MEDICINAL PLANTS OF INDIA AND CEYLON

Their chemistry and pharmacology

MEDICINAL PLANTS OF INDIA AND CEYLON

Their chemistry and pharmacology

by:
J. P. C CHANDRASENA
D.I.C., ph.D. (LOND)., A.I.C.,
Professor of Chemistry,
University College, Colombo,
Ceylon

ASIATIC PUBLISHING HOUSE
B-181/4, J-Extn, Street No-5, Laxmi-Nagar,
Delhi-110092 (**India**) Ph: (011) 2244904

ISBN 81-87067-51-9

INDIAN PRINT EDITION 2005

Printed by :
Ruchika Printers
Shahdara, Delhi-110032

Printed and Bound in India

PUBLISHER'S NOTE.

The typescript of this book had been completed, and was ready for publication when my husband, Professor J. P. C. Chandrasena, died suddenly on 10th June, 1934.

As may be seen from the contents, he has collected a large amount of material which should be useful to research workers in Chemistry and Pharmacology. References have been made to original papers, abstracts and other works of various authors. For purposes of comparison, he has extended his studies and observations to allied plants which are not found in Ceylon and India. Besides, the book gives a short account of the therapeutic properties claimed for the plants by Ayurvedic and other systems of Eastern Medicine. It should therefore be useful to those engaged in the investigation of drugs and their properties.

Being at the time of his death in charge of the teaching of Organic Chemistry at the Ceylon University College, Colombo, my husband took a great interest in this branch of his studies. During 1920 to 1922, he obtained a training in research work under Professor J. F. Thorpe, of the Royal College of Science, London. At the hands of Professor W. Straub, during 1927 to 1928, he underwent training in Pharmacology. He was also at the Imperial Institute, London, engaged in the study of drugs.

As has been stated, in the preparation of this book, resort has been made to the works of other authors. My husband's indebtedness to them, which he has not lived to acknowledge personally, must be considerable. Those authors, and their publishers, have granted their kind permission to make extracts from their works, and I take this opportunity to thank Doctors Gildemeister and Hoffmann, authors of The Volatile Oils, published by Messrs. Schimmel & Co., of Miltitz bei Leipzig, Germany; Mrs. Lewkowitsch, the representative of the late Dr. Lewkowitsch, M.A., F.I.C., author of Oils, Fats and Waxes, published by Messrs. Macmillan & Co., Ltd., London; and Dr. T. A. Henry, author of Plant Alkaloids, published by Messrs. J. & A. Churchill, Ltd., London.

I have also to acknowledge with thanks the references made by my late husband to the work by the late Dr. John Attygalle, Sinhalese Materia Medica, published in 1917, and to the Pharmacographia Indica, both now out of print.

Readers of this book will realise the difficulties necessarily experienced in publishing, in the absence of its author, a book the subject-matter of which is beyond the ken of those without a special scientific training. Constructive criticism from competent quarters is, therefore, heartily welcomed.

It remains to me to express my gratitude to Mr. B. M. F. Jayaratne, my late husband's life-long friend, for the assistance he gave, and the interest he took, in getting this book through the Press; to Mr. E. L. Fonseka, M. Sc., (Lond), A. I. C., Lecturer in Chemistry, Ceylon University College, Colombo, for his kindness in reading the proofs; and to Messrs Harrisons & Crosfield, Ltd., Colombo, for the care exercised in the printing and production of this book.

LUCY CHANDRASENA.

FOREWORD

This volume is the fruit of several years of labour on the part of my late colleague and friend, Dr. J. P. C. Chandrasena. I am not competent to assess its scientific value, but I am in a position to testify to the thoroughness and devotion to the cause of scientific research which characterised his work as lecturer and professor and researcher at this College.

Dr. Chandrasena, after serving the College as lecturer from 1922, was appointed to the Chair of Chemistry in 1933 on the retirement of Professor W. N. Rae. His death, at a time when he had established himself as an able Chemist and a stimulating teacher, robbed the College of one of the most loveable and respected personalities that have been associated with it since its foundation in 1921. I cannot do better than quote the obituary notice of him published in the Journal of the Chemical Society as testimony to his general qualities. The notice was contributed by Professor W. N. Rae, whom he succeeded as Professor of Chemistry at this College. Professor Rae wrote:—"As a Chemist he was painstaking and thorough, more interested in the work he was doing than in the publication of results, although he had several papers to his credit in the Journal of the Chemical Society and the Biochemical Journal. He was an excellent teacher and was always able to interest his students in investigation. As a colleague and friend he was admirable. A man of simple tastes, he was a Buddhist who lived up to the high tenets of his faith. He was interested in social work and did much to help the unfortunate classes. By his untimely death Ceylon loses one of the best men it has produced." There can indeed be nothing but praise for his work as a teacher and for his admirable relations with both colleagues and pupils.

He had completed the present work before his death and looked forward to its publication not only from the point of view of its general interest to chemists and pharmacologists, but also from the point of view of the value which it might have as providing, if scientific investigation at all supported them, a solid scientific foundation for the claims made for plants empirically used in the indigenous systems of medicine. Much work with a similar purport has been done in India, but little, so far as I know, in Ceylon. The book should therefore attract wide interest in Ceylon, apart from its general value to scientists in the world at large. In its special reference - I mean to Ceylon - it is justifiable to regard it as the prolegomena to a complete survey and scientific analysis of the economic and medicinal plants of Ceylon.

Mrs. Chandrasena, who publishes this work by her husband, and Mr. B. M. F. Jayaratne who has done so much to assist its publication, deserve the grateful thanks of scholars for making it accessible to the scientific world. We, who were his colleagues, mourn with them the untimely loss of an able scientist whose friendship and gentle loveable spirit will always remain a precious memory.

R. MARRS,

Principal,

Ceylon University College.

CONTENTS.

MAGNOLIACEAE.

Michelia champaka, Sinh. *Sapu,* Sans. *Champaka,* Eng. *Golden or Yellow Champa,* Tam. *Sanpang.*

A tall evergreen tree ; it grows wild in Nepal, Bengal, Assam, Burma and Ceylon. It is cultivated for its yellow, sweet-scented flowers which are used for making garlands and generally in religious worship. The leaves, flowers, fruits, bark, root and seeds are used in medicine.

The leaves are applied to indolent swellings. The leaf juice is used as a vermifuge and is also given with honey to relieve colic. The flowers are astringent and diuretic. A decoction of the flowers is used in cases of dyspepsia, nausea and fevers ; it is also useful in preventing scalding in gonorrhoea and renal diseases. When beaten up or macerated in sweet oil the flowers make an excellent local application in opthalmia and in rhimitis. The root and root-bark are described as purgative and emmenagogue. The fruit is edible and the seeds yield a fixed oil which, when rubbed on the abdomen relieves flatulence. The bark, in powder or as decoction, is given in low intermittent fevers.

The flowering season in Ceylon is from mid-June to mid-October.

Essential Oils have been distilled from several species of Michelia. The Bulletin of Roure-Bertrand

Fils (1909, 1, 26) records that the perfume from Philippine champaca is stronger and sweeter than that of the Singapore, Penang or Ceylon flowers. The fragrance of the white flowers of *M.longifolia* is altogether different from that of the flowers of yellow champaka and the two oils have no constituents in common. The odour of the flowers of the mountain species *M.nilagirica* (Sinh. *Wal Sapu*) is not as delicate as champaca. A sample of oil obtained by Schimmel & Co. (Schimmel's Reports, 1907, 6, 33,) by distilling a mixture of the white *M.longifolia* and the yellow champaka contained 60% of linalool and also methyleugenol and an ester of methyl-ethyl-acetic acid. Brooks (J. Am. Chem. Soc. 1911, 33, 1763), has found that these substances are not present in the oil from the yellow flowers. Bacon (Philippine Journal of Science, 1910, 5, 257) has, however, found 3% of iso-eugeneol in the yellow champaka oil.

Brooks (J. Am. Chem. Soc. 1911, 33, 1763) has made a chemical investigation of the essential oils of *M.champaka* and *M.longifolia.* The oil resinifies quickly on standing but treatment with sodium bisulphite slightly diminishes this tendency. The two most important constituents isolated were phenylethyl alcohol and cineole, the fine quality of the oil being due to the presence of the former, both free and as ester. On standing champaka oil deposits a large amount of a crystalline ketone (m. p. 165-166°), empirical formula $C_{16}H_{20}O_5$ $[\alpha]_D^{30°}$ – 82. 5°, (in alcohol), and yields a phenylhydrazone m. p. 161°. The oil from (white) flowers of *M.longifolia* did not give this ketone. Both the oils contain an energetic oxidase. Other constituents are isoeugeneol, benzaldehyde, benzyl alcohol and benzoic and acetic acids. The most characteristic compound in the oil from *M.longifolia* is the methyl or ethyl ester of methyl-ethyl-acetic acid.

Michelia fuscata is a very small tree and its flowers are, in the opinion of some, the most fragrant of the flowers of Ceylon.

When boiled with water, the flowers yield a yellow dye which is sometimes used as a base for other colours. They communicate an agreeable perfume to the fabric. In the Gazeteer of Orissa the bark is described as stimulant, expectorant and astringent ; the seeds and fruit are said to be useful for healing cracks in the feet and the root is described as purgative. The tincture of the flowers is much more efficient than their decoction (Watt).

ANONACEAE.

Anona squamosa, Eng. *Custard apple, sugar apple, sweet sop,* Sinh. *Anona,* Sans. *Gandhagatra, Shubha, Suda.* Tam. *Sitapalam.*

It is a native of tropical America, introduced early to the East. The principal seasons for the fruit in Ceylon are April and October. It is cultivated in Ceylon and all over India, thriving best in Cawnpore.

The leaves, seeds, and the immature fruit are largely used in some parts of India for pediculi. The leaves are also anthelmintic. The root is regarded as diuretic but is seldom, if ever, used as such.

Other species of Anonaceae are cultivated in Ceylon for the sake of the fruit but are not used in medicine.

Anona muricata, Eng. *Sour sop,* Sinh. *Katu Aththa,* Tam. *Seetha.*

Anona cherimolia, Eng. *Cherimoyer,* (no Sinhalese name), is a native of Peru, introduced into Ceylon about 1880. The fruit ripens chiefly in June-July and October-December.

Anona reticulata, Eng. *Bullocks Heart,* Sinh. *Wali Aththa* Tam. *Ramsita.*

There is a superstition among some in Ceylon that the fruit causes leprosy. The belief is perhaps due to the colour and general appearance of the rind.

BROMELIACEAE.

Ananas sativus. Eng. *Pine apple,* Sinh. *Annasi,* Tam. *Anasaphalam,* is a native of tropical America, introduced into all tropical countries.

When ripe the fruit is a most delicious table fruit. The fresh juice of the leaves is a powerful anthelmintic and vermicide ; given with sugar it relieves hiccup and also acts as a purgative. The juice of the ripe fruit contains a proteolytic enzyme and allays gastric irritability in fever ; it is also antiscorbutic. The juice of the unripe fruit in large quantities causes uterine contractions and ought to be rigorously avoided by pregnant women.

PASSIFLORACEAE.

Carica papaya, Eng. *Papaw, papaya, papeta, tree melon,* Sinh. *Pepol,* Tam. *Pappali,* is believed to be native of the shores of the Gulf of Mexico and of the West Indies and doubtfully of Brazil. All the other species of the genus are unquestionably American.

It is regarded medicinally as a remedy for haemoptysis, bleeding piles and ulcers of the urinary organs. The milk juice is used to remove warts and is also regarded as anthelmintic. It has also been used in the treatment of spleenic and hepatic enlargements. It is used as an application for ringworm and is said to be a certain remedy for scorpion bites.

Papain or Papayotin is extracted by making shallow incisions with a bone knife or a wooden splinter in the mature but still unripe fruit. The juice is collected and spread on glass to dry in the sun or in a hot-air chamber, the optimum temperature being 38°C. The time taken should not exceed 24 hours. The name " papain " is usually restricted to the pure ferment associated with a protein substance and is obtained by precipitation with alcohol and separation of albuminous matter by basic lead acetate. It is used instead of pepsin from which it differs by being active both in neutral and alkaline media. It acts not only upon muscular fibre but also upon connective tissue ; hence its use to render beef tender. For this purpose the unripe fruit is split open and rubbed over the surface of the meat before cooking. When injected into the circulation in large doses, papain paralyses the heart. In smaller quantities it appears to favour the multiplication of micrococci in the blood.

Würtz (Compt. rend., 1881, 91, 787; Abst., 1881, 750) made quantitative examinations of the digestive power of the enzyme. The seeds have been studied by Pecholt (Pharm. J. Trans. (3), 10, 343 & 383; Abst. 1880, 128) and found that they contained an oil, papaya oil; caricin, an oil-like substance with a disagreeable taste and smell, soluble in ether and alcohol; carica fat acid, an acid similar to palmitic acid; a crystalline acid, papayic acid, soluble in alcohol, insoluble in cold but soluble in hot water ; a resin acid, having an irritating and bitter taste, insoluble in water and ether but soluble in alcohol and alkalis; and a soft resin similar to that found in the fruit flesh of the "mamao femea," the fruit-bearing variety of the papaw. The leaves contain the alkaloid Carpaine to which Van Ryn assigned the formula $C_{14}H_{25}O_2N$. It has been investigated by Barger (J. Chem. Soc. 1910, 97, 466) who finds that the young leaves yield 3 to 4 times more alkaloid than mature ones. The substance crystallises in monoclinic prisms, m.p. 21°, b.p. 215-235° in vacuo, $[\alpha]_D 21°55'$ in alcohol, insoluble in water but soluble in most organic solvents. He suggests the formula

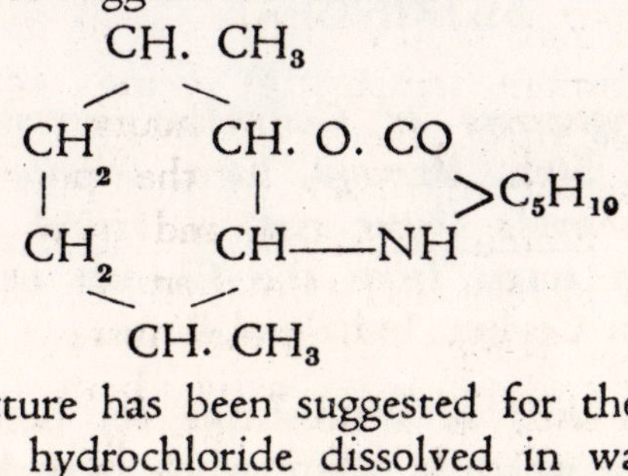

No structure has been suggested for the group C_5H_{10} Carpaine hydrochloride dissolved in water and given hypodermically (1/30 to 1/15 of a grain) can be used as a cardiac tonic in place of digitalis.

SAMYDACEAE.

Casearia esculenta. Eng. *Wild cowrie fruit,* Sinh. *Wal Waraka* Sans. *Sataganda,* Tam. *Kadlashingi,* a shrub or small tree, common in Ceylon and also found in Malabar and from Bombay to Coorg.

The root is an internal remedy for hepatic enlargement and for piles: it relieves the weight and tension in the hepatic region. It is also used in diabetes and acts as a purgative. The leaves are edible.

The bark is said to contain tannin and a substance allied to cathartic acid and the root to contain a brownish-yellow resin, a colouring matter, a small quantity of starch and an (unidentified) neutral substance. crystallizing in white transparent prisms.

OCHNACEAE.

Ochna squarrosa. Sinh. *Mal keera,* Tam. *Chilanki.*

Ochna wightiana. Sinh. *Bo keera,* Tam. *Katkari.*

Both these are said to be used in medicine.

MORINGEAE.

Moringa pterygosperma or Guilandina moringa or Hyperanthea moringa, Sinh. *Murunga,* Sans. *Sobanjana, Dvishigru, Murungi, Danshamula (bitter root)* is found wild in the sub-Himalayan tracts from the Chenab to Oudh, and is cultivated in Ceylon, India and Burma.

The root is used as a substitute for horse-radish. It yields a gum, which is white when fresh but gradually turns to a mahogany colour on keeping. On account of this dark colour, the gum is of no commercial value.

The seeds yield a clear, limpid, almost colourless oil which is easily extracted by pressure. Both this and the oil from *M.aptera* are commercially termed Ben or Beni Oil (not made in Ceylon and seldom in India) and are used as lubricants by watch makers. Walter obtained from the oil of *M.aptera* an acid which he called Moringic Acid but which Zaleski later (Ber., 1874, 7, 1013) proved to be identical with oleic acid. The root bark, with the leaves of *Rumex vesicarius,* (Sans. *Chukra*) black and long pepper, and rock salt, made into a decoction, is given in ascites and enlarged spleen. Externally the decoction of the root bark is used to foment inflamed parts, to relieve spasms or it is applied to the inflamed part as a plaster. In Bengal it is believed that half-ounce doses of the bark cause abortion. The fresh juice of the leaves, when poured into the ear, relieves otalgia, it also relieves dental caries. The pods act as a preventive against intestinal worms. The seeds are said to be stimulant. The leaf juice is used as an emetic. A poultice of the leaves is useful in relieving glandular swellings, but it has the disadvantage of always producing blisters.

The bark is said to contain a white crystalline alkaloid, two resins, an inorganic acid and mucilage. The root has been examined by Broughton who obtained from it, by steam distillation, an essential oil of " disgusting " odour and much pungency. It differs from the oil of mustard and garlic, the odour being distinct and more offensive (Watt, V, 278).

Lewkowitsch (Vol. II, page 381-384, 1922 Edition) gives an account of Ben Oil. Northern Nigerian *Moringa* seeds submitted to him by The Imperial Institute contained 33.27% oil. The seeds consisted of 92% of kernel. They were expressed in two stages on a semi-large scale, and yielded a cold-pressed and a hot-pressed oil, which gave the following values :—

	Cold-pressed crude Ben oil.	Hot-pressed crude oil.
Sp. Gr. at 40° ..	0.9018	0.8984
Acid Value ..	49.71	100.5
Sap. Value ..	179.2	178.7
Unsap. matter ..	1.67%	2.69%
Iodine value ..	100.3	88
Titer test of fatty acids ..	32°C	38.2°C

The oil has a slightly yellowish colour, is inodorous and has a sweet taste. The phytosterol isolated by van Italie and Nieuwland melted at 131-135°.

On the strength of experiments made in Jamaica in 1817, Ben oil was considered extremely valuable for delicate machinery, and was credited with the property of not readily turning rancid. Lewkowitsch's experiments, however, show this assumption to be erroneous; the oil becomes rancid just like any other oil, the rancidity depending on the manner in which it has been kept. He further states that if properly refined, it would be a good edible one and would also be a valuable lubricant for delicate machinery. (See also Lewkowitsch, Analyst 1903, 343).

The composition of the cakes has been examined. (Bull. Imp. Inst., 1908, 361.)

NYMPHAEACEAE

The *nymphaeaceae* are aquatic herbs, usually floating. The flowers have numerous petals and very numerous stamens. There are two species :—*Nymphaea*, having seeds with endosperm and *Nelumbium*, having seeds without endosperm.

Nelumbium speciosum. Eng. *Lotus,* Sinh. *Nelum,* Sans. *Padma, Kamal,* Tam. *Tamarai.*

The flowers have received a great deal of attention in the literature and religion of India and other countries.

The stalks yield a fibre. It is said that the viscid juice of the leaf and flower stalks is a remedy in diarrhoea and that the petals are slightly astringent. The root in the form of a paste is employed in ringworm and other cutaneous affections. The filaments are astringent and cooling and prescribed for burning sensation of the body, bleeding from piles and menorrhagia. The seeds are used to check vomiting and are also given to children as diuretic and refrigerant. The various parts of the herb form an ingredient in many decoctions.

Nymphaea. Eng. *Lotus.* Sinh. *Olu, or Atholu,* Sans. *Kumuda,* Tam. *Ampal.*

The fruit is edible. The flower is used as a dry and cold astringent in diarrhoea, cholera, fever and diseases of the liver and is also recommended as a cardiac tonic. The powdered root is prescribed for piles as a demulcent, also for dysentery and dyspepsia. The seeds are a cooling medicine for cutaneous diseases and leprosy and are considered as antidote for poisons.

Nymphaea stellata. Sinh. *Manel,* Sans. *Nilotphala.*

The *nymphaeae* have been investigated by Gruning (Abst. 1883, 369). He examined *N.alba* which was a very popular remedy in Germany at one time. He made various extracts of the rhizomes and isolated an alkaloid which Dragendorff had previously isolated in 1879. Tannins are also found which yield many secondary products which have been found in other tannins.

OLACINEAE.

Olax zeylanica. Sinh. *Mella.*

This is a small shrub indigenous to Ceylon and common in low-lying parts. Its leaves are used as salad, and fried with red onions and ghee are eaten for frequent and painful micturition.

CRASSULACEAE.

Kalanchoe laciniata. Sinh. *Akkapana,* Tam. *Mala-kulli,* Sans. *Hamasagara, Parnavija, Asthibaksha.* The last two Sanskrit names mean " leaf-seed," because their leaves, when placed upon moist ground, take root and produce young plants. It is a native of Tropical Africa and grows wild in Bengal, Deccan and Ceylon.

The leaves are styptic, astringent and antiseptic, and form an excellent application for wounds and contusions as they allay inflammation and swelling, and prevent discolouration and heal the wound rapidly. The juice of leaves is given with butter in diarrhoea, dysentery, cholera and phthisis.

MELASTOMACEAE.

Memecylon edule vel tinctorium. Sinh. *Dadikaha, Walikaha,* Sans. *Anjane,* Tam. *Kashamaram,* Eng. *The iron wood tree.*

This tree is remarkable for its bright green foliage and clusters of purplish, blue flowers. The leaves yield a yellow dye which is a glucoside. This dye is employed in South India for dyeing a " delicate yellow lake " and, in conjunction with myrobalans and sappan wood, the leaves produce a deep red tinge much used for dyeing grass mats and cloth. In medicine, the leaves have been found to be a remedy of considerable reputation for gonorrhoea in Belgium. They are cooling and astringent and are used in diarrhoea and dysentery. A 1 in 20 infusion of the leaves in used as a collyrium in conjunctivitis. The roots in decoction are used in excessive menstrual discharge.

CACTACEAE.

Opuntia Dillenii, (Cactus indicus). Eng. *The prickly pear,* Sinh. *Katupatuk,* Sans. *Vidara-visva,* Tam. *Nagar kali, Naga-dali.*

A native of America (Brazil), introduced into the East by the Portuguese for feeding the cochineal insect and is now quite naturalized in India and Ceylon.

The fruit is edible and can be employed in the distillation of alcohol. The fibre is used in India for the manufacture of paper. Hooper's Analysis (Watt) of the fruit from Nellore gives carbohydrates 4.89%, fibre 32%, albuminoids 6.25%, fats 3.63%, water 5.67%, ash 10.56%.

The fruit is refrigerant and its syrup acts as an expectorant, hence its use in whooping-cough, asthma and spasmodic cough ; it is also used in hepatic congestion. It has been used by Western practitioners in the treatment of heart disease.

The mucilage obtained from the plant consists chiefly of galactan (Abst. 1896, 11, 60), and according to Harlay, (Abst. 1902, 11, 685) the mucilage from *Opuntia vulgaris* consists for the most part of araban and galactan : the solution is dextro-rotatory.

CAMPANULACEAE.

Lobelia nicotianaefolia. Sinh. *Rasni, Waldunkola, (wild tobacco);* Sans. *Dhabala,;* Tam. *Kattu-poillai.* The wild variety which is known as Kiribamboo, is used in Ceylon Up-country estates as a protection against " black grub " or " cut-worm." Its chief value is as a remedy for asthma. It is used less in Ceylon than in India. The dry herb and seeds are said to be extremely acrid and the dust of the former irritates the throat and nostrils like tobacco, hence the Sinhalese and Tamil names. It is also said that the seeds contain an acro-narcotic poison and that they are preferred to *Datura* as a poison when rapid action is required. It is, in fact, more widely known as a poison than as a drug.

PRIMULACEAE.

Cylclamen indicum. Sans. *Talamule,* Sinh. *Oorala.*

It is frequently used with other drugs and is regarded as very useful in Wataṛakta ("Burning" of the feet).

MYRSINEAE.

Embelia Ribes. Sinh. *Wel-embilla,* Sans. *Vidanga, Vrisha-nasana* ; Tam. *Vayu-vilangam.*

It is different from *Wel-embiliya,* or *Rata-embiliya,* which is *Elaeagnus latifolia* (*Elaeagnaceae*), of no therapeutic value.

The berries, leaves and root-bark are used in medicine.

Embelic acid, $C_9H_{14}O_2$, was isolated by Warden (Abst. 1889, 1, 408) from an alcoholic extract in the form of crystals, insoluble in water, m.p. 140°, decomposing at 155°, with partial sublimation. The ammonium salt was found effective as an anthelmintic for taenia ; it has the advantage of being tasteless. See also Heyl and Kneip, (Abst. 1913, ii, 1083.) Embelic acid is the substance to which the anthelmintic action of the plant is due.

An alkaloid, christembine, also appears to have been isolated.

The dried berries, sold in the Ceylon bazaars as *Valangasal,* are used for their carminative, anthelmintic, stimulant and alterative action. For expelling worms the powdered seed is given in 60 grain doses. The berries are also used in many decoctions for fevers and diseases of the skin and chest. It is a common practice in the neighbourhood of Bombay to put a few of the berries in the milk that is given to young children to prevent flatulence.

The fresh juice of the leaves is cooling, diuretic and laxative and the pulp is purgative. The drug enters into the composition of several applications for ringworm and other skin diseases.

Vidanga Taila, which is used for relieving headache or hemicrania by rubbing it on the forehead or dropping it in the nose, is composed of *Embelia ribes, Croton tiglium* and sodium carbonate.

EBENACEAE.

Diospyros embryopteris. Sinh. *Timbiri,* Sans. *Tinduka,* Tam. *Tumbilik-kai,* is a dense ever-green, small tree with dark-green foliage and long shining leaves, common throughout India and Burma.

The fruit, the bark and the gummy exudation are very astringent. In Bengal, a preparation made by heating the fruit in a large mortar, and boiling the expressed juice and mixing with powdered charcoal, is applied to planks. A brownish liquid used for dyeing and tanning is prepared from the half-ripe fruit. In Ceylon, the plant is used for dyeing fishnets, for preventing decay, and also in caulking boats as a protection against insects.

The ripe fruit is edible and is beneficial in blood diseases and in gonorrhoea and leprosy. In India "*Tunika Oil*" obtained from the seeds is used in dysentery and diarrhoea. Although the ripe fruit is very sweet insects will not touch it. An infusion or decoction of the rind is useful in chronic dysentery and diarrhoea.

Hummel has found that the fruit contains 15% tannic acid. It is recorded that the testa are the most astringent part of the seed. It would be very instructive to have the fruit chemically examined in all its stages of growth. The properties ascribed to it in the literature both as a drug and as a tar, seem to be founded on imperfect material.

Considerable confusion also exists on the subject of the gum or resin obtained from the tree ; it ought to be further investigated.

PORTULACEAE.

Portulaca oleracea, the Common Indian *Purslane,* Sinh. *Genda,* Sans. *Lonika, Lonamla,* Tam. *Puli-kerai* and *P.quadrifida,* Sinh. *Heen-genda,* Sans. *Laghu lonika,* Tam. *Parpukirai,* are abandant weeds in cultivated ground, found throughout India.

They are diuretic and febrifuge and have been long used in India and Ceylon as a domestic remedy. The plants and the seeds are used in kidney and bladder diseases such as dysuria, haematuria and gonorrhoea, and are also praised as an application in burns, scalds and various forms of skin disease. The herbs give a large quantity of a milky juice which is used in cases of gonorrhoea and scanty urine. The seeds are beneficial to the intestinal mucous membrane and are therefore useful in dysentery. The bruised fresh leaves, which are acid, are prescribed as an external application in erysipelas and an infusion of them is given as a diuretic. In Jamaica, it is employed as a cooling and moistening herb in burning fevers. The fresh succulent leaves are recommended as a cooling external application.

Storer and Lewis (Abst. 1879, 821) have analysed *Portulaca* collected in July and have found that the fresh leaves are rich in protein (2.2%.)

GERANIACEAE.

Oxalis corniculata, Indian Sorrell, Sinh. *Embul-embiliya, Heen-embul-embiliya,* Sans. *Amla-lonika, Changeri,* Tam. *Puliyarai.*

A very common garden weed, abundant throughout the warmer parts of India and Ceylon. Its acid taste is due to the presence of potassium hydrogen oxalate.

It is regarded as a tonic; it is antiscorbutic, astringent, stomachic and useful in fevers and biliousness. The fresh leaves made into a curry improve the appetite of dyspeptics. The fresh juice is given to relieve intoxication from *Datura* and is said to be useful in dysentery and prolapsus of the rectum. Chakradatta recommends his "*Changeri Ghrita*" for diarrhoea, dysentery, prolapsus of the rectum and difficult micturition. It is made in the usual way from clarified butter 4 seers, fresh juice of *O. corniculata* 4 seers, and leaves of the same reduced to a paste, 4 seers.

The following plants of this natural order, although not mentioned in the *Nigandhus*, are occasionally used in medicine :— *Biophytum sensitivum*, Sinh. *Gas-nidikumba*; *Impatiens repens*, Sinh. *Galdemata*; *Hydrocera augustifolia*, Sinh. *Diya-koodalu*; *Averrhoa carambola*, Sinh. *Karamba* or *Kamaranga*; *A.Bilimbi*, Sinh. *Billing*, Tam. *Pulusakalalu*.

Averrhoa bilimbi is cultivated for its cylindrical fruit about 2" long, which is very sour when green but loses some of its acidity when ripe. The fruits are generally used in pickle and in curry. The flowers are made into preserves.

Averrhoa carambola is a small tree with sensitive leaflets. The unripe apples are astringent and are used as an acid in dyeing, the acid probably acting as a mordant. The leaves, the fruit and the root are used as cooling medicines. The acid, dried fruit is given in fevers ; it has anti-scorbutic properties.

LINACEAE.

Erythroxylon acidum. Sinh. *Batakirilla*, Tam. *Chiruchemannathi*,—is a much-branched twiggy shrub found in the low country of Ceylon and occurs as an undergrowth in forests.

It is the best and most effective anthelmintic in Sinhalese medicine. It is given in various forms : the usual one is to mix the powdered dry leaves with flour and honey and make into " aggala " or large-sized pills.

Erythroxylon monogynum, Bastard Sandal or Red Cedar, has no Sinhalese name but the Tamils call it *Thevatharan* or *Chemmanatti* on account of the fragrance of its wood and leaves. Its heartwood is very hard, smooth and dark-brown. It has a pleasant resinous scent and yields, on distillation, a kind of oil resembling tar, which is used as a preservative for the wood of boats. This oily substance is known to the Sinhalese as *Dummela*. It is soluble in ether, alcohol and turpentine. It has not hitherto been a commercial article.

It is said that during the Madras famine of 1877, the leaves were largely eaten by the starving poor. It seemed probable that the leaves contain some principle like that of *E.coca*, that is cocaine. Specimens analysed in Madras, however, were found to have no anaesthetic property but to possess a bitter and tonic alkaloid which might mitigate the pangs of hunger. Another chemical examination carried out by Waddell confirmed this result (Pharm. Indica).

The plant is described as possessing stomachic, diaphoretic and stimulant-diuretic properties.

Erythroxylon coca (*cocaine*) is not a native of Ceylon and its cultivation has been prohibited.

ZYGOPHYLLEAE.

Tribulus terrestris. (*Small caltrops*), Sinh. *Sembu-nerenchi*, Sans. *Gokshuri*, or *Ikshugandha*, Tam. *Nerenji-kirai*, is a low trailing annual plant, common in sandy soil throughout India and Ceylon.

The fruit and root are used in medicine and form an ingredient of many important decoctions, among them the *Dasamula* or Ten Root decoction.

The drug has been used in cases of Bright's disease with success (Indigenous Drugs Report, Madras). Water rendered mucilaginous by the plant is drunk as a remedy for impotence caused by malpractices or old age ; it is also given with sesamum seed and goat's milk for the same condition. The decoction of the fruits with the addition of potassium carbonate is given for painful micturition (Chakradatta).

Pharmacographia Indica mentions that the fruit contains a body having the properties of an alkaloid and associated with hydrochloric acid or alkali chloride, and that it yields a fat and a resin, the latter when burned is fragrant.

The ten plants, the roots of which go to form the *Dasamula Kvatha* are: *Desmodium gangeticum, Uraria lagopodioides, Solanum Jacquini, Tribulus terrestris, Aegle Marmelos, Calosanthes indica, Gmelina arborea, Stereospermum suaveolens, and Premna spinosa.* The first five are called *Hrasva* or *Laghu Pancha Mula* (the five minor roots), and the last. five *Vrihat Pancha Mula* (the five major roots).

ONAGRACEAE.

Jussiaea suffructicosa. Sinh. *Bera-diyamilla,* Sans. *Bhalla-vianga, Bhalavaanga,* Tam. *Neer-kirambu.*

A perennial undershrub found all over India and Ceylon. It is regarded as a powerful astringent. The plant ground fine and steeped in butter-milk is considered useful in diarrhoea and dysentery. Its decoction is used to dissipate flatulence, to increase urine and as a purgative and anthelmintic.

PAPAVERACEAE.

No plants of this natural order are found in Ceylon but opium (Sinh. *Abin*) is a common drug in Ayurvedic medicine.

CRUCIFERAE

Sinapis alba. Eng. *White Mustard,* Sinh. *Ela-aba;* Sans. *Svetasarisha, Siddhartha;* Tam. *Venkadaku.*

Mustard flour is nervine, stimulant, emetic and diuretic. In small doses it promotes digestion and removes flatus. In large doses it is stimulant-emetic and narcotic-poison when given with hot water. The volatile oil is stimulant, rubefacient and vesicant.

Brassica campestria, Eng. *Rape seed,* Sinh. *Wal-aba;* Sans. *Sarshapa;* or *Rakthasarshapa.*

The seed gives an oil which is rubefacient and is used in skin disease.

Brassica nigra, Eng. *Black or true Mustard,* Sinh. *Kalu-aba;* Sans. *Asuri;* Tam. *Chirukaduku.*

Externally the seed oil is stimulant and mild counter-irritant. Internally the seeds are emetic. In moderate doses they are digestive and laxative. The leaves are pungent and stomachic.

The volatile oil does not exist ready formed in the seeds, but is a product of the action of the enzyme Myrosin on sinigrin (potassium myronate). When the seeds are dry these bodies do not come in contact, but directly water is added, the myrosin decomposes the sinigrin in the seed.

Brassica Juncea, Eng. *Indian Mustard,* Sinh. *Aba;* Sans. *Sarshapa, Rajika;* Tam. *Kaduku.*

This is a tall, erect, annual tree, cultivated abundantly in India and extends westward to Egypt and eastward to China. This is the plant which in India bears the name of mustard and takes the place of *B. nigra* in all warm countries.

It is used more as a condiment than as a medicine. It is the basic ingredient of the well-known medicinal oil, *Siddhartha Taila,* used as an external application for all rheumatic and other pains and in cases of oppression, followed usually by immediate relief. In infantile convulsions, a few drops are poured into the ears and a drop or two is even given internally.

For external use the seeds, when combined with *moringa* bark or garlic are more active than when used alone.

Schimmel & Co. (Abst. 1910, 1, 759) have found the following constants for a specimen of essential oil prepared from Indian mustard:— $D_{15°}$ 0.9950,$[\alpha]_D$ + 0° 12' $n_D^{20°}$ 1.51849, b.p. 150-160° and 174-178°. The principal constituents are dimethyl sulphide, allyl cyanide, allyl thiocarbimide and a crotonylthiocarbamide.

From *Sinapis Alba,* Will and Laubenheimer (Ann. 1879, *199*, 150; Abst. 1880, 265) isolated a glucoside, *Sinalbin,* $C_{80}H_{44}N_2S_2O_{16}$, by extracting the seeds with warm alcohol, after previously removing the fixed oil by pressure and treatment with carbon disulphide. It crystallised from dilute alcohol and the mother liquor contained sinapin thiocyanate. By extraction with water the enzyme, myrosin, was also prepared, which decomposes sinalbin to sinalbin thiocarbimide, sinapin sulphate and sugar.

Remsen and Coale (Am. Chem. J. 1884, 6, 50; Abst. 1884, 1387) describe a method for preparing Sinapine thiocyanate, m.p. 176°. Sinapic acid, $C_{11}H_{12}O_5$, m.p. 185-192° was also isolated.

The composition of *Sinapis alba* during various stages of growth has been investigated by Hornberger (Landwirtschaft. Versuchs-Stat. 1885, 415; Abst. 1885, 1087).

The glucosides of black and white mustards have been investigated by Gadamer (Abst. 1897, 1, 254, 360). He isolated pot ssium myronate (sinigrin) $C_{10}H_{16}NS_2O_9K$, m.p. 126-127a $[\alpha]_D-15.2°$. Air dried sinalbin, the glucoside of white mustard, has the composition $C_{30}H_{42}N_2S_2O_{15}$ 5 H_2O, m. p. 83-84°. In the presence of myrosin this combines with water and yields an essential oil, $C_7H_7O.NCS$, sinapin hydrogen sulphate and d-glucose. See also Gadamer, (Ber. 1897, *30*, 2322) and for the migration of Nitrogenous Substances and Ternary substances in *Sinapis alba,* Andre, (Compt. rend. 1901, *132*, 1058; Abst. 1901, ii, 413).

For the Synthesis of Sinapic Acid see Graebe & Martz, (Ber. 1903, *36*, 1031; Abst. 1903, I, 492) and for the Synthesis of Sinapin, (Spath, Monatsh. 1920, *41*, 271; Abst. 1921, 1, 28).

Lepidium sativum, Eng. *Water cress*, Sans. *Chandra-suriya;* Tam. *Alivirai,*— is the garden cress of Europe andi s cultivated as a vegetable in Asia also.

The seeds are aperient, diuretic, alterative, tonic and aphrodisiac. They are given with mucilage for hiccup and for the dispersion of chronic enlargements of the spleen. It is an ingredient in preparations for various diseases.

Gadamer (Ber. 1899, *32*, 2335; Abst. 1899. i, 930) finds that the essential oil from the seeds of *L. sativum* consists principally of benzylthiocarbimide mixed with variable quantities of benzyl cyanide; both are produced by the decomposition of a glucoside, the former by the action of myrosin and the latter by the action of boiling water and acids. The glucoside itself was not obtained in the crystalline form. (See also A. W. Hofmann, Ber. 1874, 7, 1293.)

The fatty oil of cress seeds is brownish-yellow in colour and has the following properties:—sp. gr. 0.924, thickens and becomes turbid at 6-10° and congeals at 15° to a yellow mass, has a peculiar smell and taste and dries slowly (Schubler).

Raphanus sativus. Sinh. *Rabu;* Sans. *Moolaka;* Tam. *Mullangi,*— is the common garden radish and is largely cultivated all over India and Ceylon.

The seeds and leaves are diuretic, laxative and lithontriptic. The seeds are also believed to have emmenagogue properties. The root is a reputed medicine for haemorrhoids and is also given in urinary and syphilitic complaints to relieve dysuria and strangury. It is also powerfully antiscorbutic.

Moreigne (Abst. 1897, 1, 94) isolated from the aqueous extract of the root of *Raphanus niger*, a crystalline substance, raphanol, $C_{29}H_{58}O_4$, m.p. 62°, probably a polyhydroxy-lactone.

CAPPARIDEAE

Crataeva religiosa vel Roxburghii, Sinh. *Lunuwaruna;* Sans. *Varuna, Pashuganda Asmarighna (asmari — gravel or stone);* Tam. *Mavihankai;* Eng. *Holy garlic pear.*

As one of the Sanskrit names implies, the plant is used on account of its lithontriptic action; for this purpose the root and the bark are used. The root is also alterative. A very efficacious decoction is made of gokatu (*Tribulus terrestris*), ginger and *C. religiosa* in equal quantities; this is a very effectve lithontriptic. The fresh leaves are, externally, rubefacient and internally febrifuge and tonic. They are also used in the form of decoction for swelling and for burning sensation in the feet, a condition described in Ayurveda as Raktha Vatha.

Capparis horrida, Sinh. *Welangiriya;* Sans. *Ardanda;* Tam. *Kilacchedi,*— is a climbing thorny shrub growing in most parts of India and Burma and in the hot dry tracts of Ceylon.

Capparis zeylancia, Sans. *Karira*— is a variety of above, for which *Capparis Spinosa* is used, a species growing in the deserts of Rajputana, Punjab and Sindh.

The two plants are not much used in medicine. The green fruit is cooked and eaten. The leaves are applied as counter-irritant. The bark, along with native spirit, is given in cholera. In Madras, a decoction of the leaves is used in syphilis.

Wachs (Abst. 1894, i, 299) investigated the yellow colouring matters of the flower buds of *C. spinosa*. (See Watts Dict. of Chem.) These yield, on hydrolysis, compounds of the formula $C_{15}H_{10}O_7$ which are identical or isomeric with quercetin, and also glucose and isodulcitol.

Wunderlich (Abst. 1908, i, 559) isolated a rhamnoside identical with rutin, obtained from rue.

Molisch (Abst. 1917, i, 505) has found micro-chemically in the leaf stem of *C. callosa* a spherical, colourless, highly refractive body which is an organic calcium compound, possibly a double malate of calcium and magnesium. These two bodies are also found in the leaf and the stem.

Cleome viscosa, Sinh. *Wal-aba*, ; Sans. *Aditiyabhakta* or *Arkabhakta* ; Tam. *Naivela*.

An annual weed from 1-3 feet high. It has a powerful odour like black currants, the leaves have a pungent flavour and the seeds a feeble taste of mustard. The juice of the leaves is poured into the ear to relieve ear-ache. The Pharmacopoeia Indica states that the juice mixed with oil is a popular remedy in Bombay for purulent discharges from the ear. The leaves boiled in ghee are applied to recent wounds and the juice to ulcers.

The seeds are anthelmintic, rubefacient and vesicant and are useful in expelling round worms. When subjected to great pressure, the seeds yield a light olive-green, limpid oil. "It seems likely that this oil would prove serviceable when a very liquid oil is required."

Gynandropsis pentaphylla, Sinh. *Wela;* Sans. *Arkapushpika;* *Tam. Taiwela.*

A small annual herb abundant throughout warmer parts of India and all tropical countries.

The seeds are anti-spasmodic, sudorific, anthelmintic and carminative. In powder they are given internally for two days for the expulsion of round worms, followed by castor oil on the third day. The juice of the leaves is used as an anodyne instillation for relief of pain in otalgia and catarrahal inflammation of the middle ear. The leaves are applied to boils to prevent the formation of pus.

Attygalle (page 18) records a curious prescription for severe colic :—" Pound *wela* well in a mortar, mix the juice with human milk and pour into the ear for severe colic."

The seeds rubbed up with oil are used as a vermicide in dressing the hair. They are also said to be employed for poisoning fish.

BIXINEAE.

Cochlospermum Gossypium, Eng. white silk-cotton tree, Sinh. *Heeni-kiriya; Elaimbul;* Sans. *Kathira, Katira;* Tam. *Tanaku Koge.*

This is frequently found on rocky hills in the dry districts, but usually near the temples and planted for the sake of the large golden yellow flowers which are used for offerings.

The gum exuding from the plant is used immediately and is a substitute for Gum Tragacanth. Mixed with curd or whey, the gum is beneficial in diarrhoea and dysentery. The tender leaves boiled in water make a cooling hair-wash.

The chemistry of the gum has been investigated by H. H. Robinson (J. Chem. Soc. 1906, 89, 1496). It has the remarkable property of giving off acetic acid on exposure to moist air. It does not dissolve to any extent in water and is free from starch. Lemeland (J. pharm. Chim. 1904, 20, 253) had, however, previously isolated galactose. Robinson obtained a stable acid $C_{23}H_{36}O_{21}$, for which the name "gondic acid" was proposed (gond is Hindustani for gum); xylose, a hexose, α-cochlospermic acid. He also suggests that the gum itself is a tetra-acetyl derivative of the last mentioned acid, which may be a hexosan-xylosan-gondic acid.

Flacourtia Ramontchi, Mauritius Plum, Flacourtia; Sinh. *Uguressa;* Sans. *Vikarigata, Svadukantaka;* Tam. *Katukuli.*

A small tree with long spinous twigs and globular edible fruit. It is seldom used in medicine. The fruit is, however, given in jaundice and enlarged spleen. The gum is administered along with other ingredients in cholera.

Flacourtia cataphracta, Many-spined Flacourtia, Sinh. *Rata-uguressa;* Sans. *Prachinamalaka;* Tam. *Shimai-katukali.* This was introduced into Ceylon from Malaya and gives a better fruit than *F. Ramontchi.*

The bark is astringent, the leaves and young shoots are stomachic; the dried leaves are carminative, stomachic, tonic and astringent. The fruit is said to be useful in bilious conditions, relieves nausea and checks vomiting. An infusion of the bark is given in hoarseness.

Scolopia Gaertneri, Sinh. *Katukurundu,* has an edible fruit like that of *F. Ramontchi.*

Gynocardia odorata, Sans. *Chaulmoogara,* is a moderate-sized ever-green, glabrous tree, readily known by the hard round fruits which grow on the stem and main branches. It is found in Sikkim and the Khasia Mts. eastward to Chittagong, Rangoon and Tenasserim.

The seeds of this plant and the nearly allied *Hydnocarpus Wightiana* have long been used as a remedy for leprosy. The seeds and oil are both largely used and are as a rule administered with ghee. They are supposed to be alterative and tonic internally, stimulant when applied externally. In 1856, *Chaulmoogra.* was brought to the notice of the Europeans in India as a remedy for secondary syphilis; later, it was described by Jones as an efficient alterative tonic in cases of phthsis and scrofula, and in 1868, it was included in the Pharmacopoeia of India.

Hydnocarpus is a genus belonging to this natural order and comprises about six species, inhabitants of Tropical Asia.

Hydnocarpus alpina, is a large tree 70-100 feet high, common on the Nilgiris up to 6,000 feet; found also in Tinnevelly and in Ceylon up to 1,500 feet. The seeds yield an oil which is employed for burning in Karwar.

Hydnocarpus heterophylla is found in Burma.

Hydnocarpus Odorata is synonymous with *Gynocardia odorata.*

Hydnocarpus Venenata is a large tree found in Ceylon, called *Makulu* in Sinhalese. It grows on the banks of rivers up to 2,000 feet. It is also found in Malabar, Tinnevelly and Travancore.

In recent years the chemical and pharmacological values of the oils derived from these plants have been carefully investigated by several investigators. In 1876, Dymock (Pharm. J. Trans. [3], vi, 761) examined the oils of *H. Wightiana* and *G.odorata*. In 1879 Moss (Year Book of Pharmacy, 1879, 522) made a chemical examination of "*chaulmoogra*" oil, probably a commercial sample. By hydrolysing the oil he obtained 81.1% of fatty acids, which were considered to consist of "gynocardic", palmitic, hypogaeic and "cocinic" acids. Petit (J. pharm. Chim., 1892, 26, 445) published a method of preparing gynocardic acid, which really was that portion of the fatty acids melting at 29°.

Schindelmeiser (Ber. deut. pharm. Ges. 1904, *14*, 164) accepted in general the conclusions of Moss, but without any confirmatory evidence.

Power and Gornall (J. Chem. Soc.,1904, *85*, 838) examined the constituents of fresh "chaulmoogra" seeds which were identified as the product of *Taraktogenos Kurzii* (King). On bruising the seeds hydrocyanic acid was liberated, presumably by the action of an enzyme present in the seeds. The kernels, freed from the shells, on complete extraction with ether gave 32.2% of fixed oil. The oil investigated was prepared by pressure. From the "presscake," the following were isolated :—a hydrolytic enzyme capable of hydrolysing amygdalin to benzaldehyde and hydrocyanic acid ; a syrupy glucoside by extraction with alcohol ; this latter extract gave a little acetic acid, a phytosterol, and an olefinic substance of the formula $C_{18}H_{32}O_2$. The fatty oil gave the following constants:—

	Expressed oil	Oil extracted by ether
M. P.	22-23°	22-23°
Sp. Gr.	0.951 at 25° 0.940 at 45°	0.952 at 25° 0.942 at 45°
$[\alpha]_D^{15°}$	+52.0°	+51.3°
Acid value	23.9	9.5
Saponification Value	213.0	208.0
Iodine value	103.2	104.4

On hydrolysis the oil yielded a phytosterol, $C_{26}H_{44}O$, m. p. 132°, glycerol, palmitic acid, and a new unsaturated acid $C_{18}H_{32}O_2$ chaulmoogric acid, m. p. 68°, $[\alpha]_D + 56°$.

At the same time, the constitution of this new acid was investigated by the same authors (J. Chem. Soc. 1904, *85*, 851) and later by Barrowcliff and Power (J. Chem. Soc. 1907, *91*, 557). The latter paper also deals with the constitution of hydnocarpic acid.

Power and Lees (J. Chem. Soc. 1907, *87*, 349) isolated a new cyanogenetic glucoside, gynocardin, from the seeds of *G. odorata*, in 5% yield. It has the formula $C_{13}H_{19}O_6N$, m. p. 163°, crystallises from water with 1½ molecules of water, $[\alpha]_D^{21°}$ + 72.5°, very stable towards the usual acid hydrolytic agents, gives a hepta-acetyl derivative, and is hydrolysed by hot baryta or acid and the enzyme in the seed. Hydrolysis with baryta gives gynocardinic acid which itself hydrolyses to glucose and an acid of unknown constitution.

Power and Barrowcliff have studied the constituents of *H. Wightiana* and *H. anthelmintica* (J. Chem. Soc. 1905, *87*, 884). These two plants have been long used in Western India and China respectively. *H. anthelmintica* is a tree indigenous to Siam, the seeds of which are exported to China under the name of Lukrabo. The fatty oils from these two species very closely resemble chaulmoogra oil (which, as has already been mentioned, is the product of *Taraktogenos Kurzii*) both in their physical characters and their chemical composition. The acids obtained from them consist chiefly of chaulmoogric acid and a lower homologue of the same series, the latter being present in both the oils and in chaulmoogra oil. The new acid, named hydnocarpic acid, $C_{16}H_{28}O_2$, crystallises from alcohol, has m. p. 60°, $[\alpha]_D + 68°$ in chloroform solution, contains only one ethylene linkage and must, therefore, contain, like chaulmoogric acid, an alicyclic group.

The seeds of *H. Wightiana* contain 41.2% of fixed oil, which has the following constants :—

	Expressed	Oil extracted by ether
M. P.	22-23°	22-23°
Sp. Gr. at 25°	0.958	0.959
$[\alpha]_D$ in Chloroform	+57.7°	+56.2°
Acid value	3.8	7.4
Saponification Value	207.0	207.0
Iodine value	101.3	102.5

By hydrolysing the oil the authors obtained a phytosterol $C_{26}H_{44}O$, m. p. 132-133°; chaulmoogric acid and hydnocarpic acid.

The oil of *H. anthelmintica* has the following constants :—

	Expressed oil	Oil extracted by ether
M. P.	24-25°	23-24°
Sp. Gr. at 25°	0.953	0.952
$[\alpha]_D$ in chloroform	52.5°	51.0
Acid value	7.5	8.1
Saponification value	212.0	208.0
Iodine value	86.4	82.5

With the object of identifying the glucoside, gynocardine, previously isolated by Power and Lees (J. Chem. Soc. 1905, 87, 349), Moore and Tutin (J. Chem. Soc. 1910, 97, 1,285) methylated it and hydrolysed the methylation product. The only conclusion, however, that they were able to draw was that the glucoside, gynocardine, and the enzyme, gynocardase belong to the β series.

De Jong (Rec. trav. chim., 1911, 30, 220; Abst. 1912, 1, 39) has found that gynocardine, on hydrolysis with the enzyme of the leaves of *Pangium edule* gives glucose, hydrogen cyanide and a substance $C_6H_8O_4$, which is a diketone and yields a phenylhydrazone which decomposes at 177°. $C_{13}H_{19}O_9N + H_2O = C_6H_{12}O_6 + HCN + C_6H_8O_4$.

Leonard Rogers (Brit. Med. J. 1916, 11, 550; Abst. 1916, 1, 860) found that the fraction of lower melting point (up to 40°) of the fatty acids of chaulmoogra oil from the seeds of *Taraktogenos Kurzi* (vide J. Chem. Soc. 1904, 85, 838, 851) is the most useful in the treatment of leprosy. This so-called gynocardic acid is best given intravenously as sodium salt. The fraction of m. p. 40.8-43°, with sodium salts scarcely soluble in water, contains chaulmoogric acid and is unsuitable for injection and, probably, therapeutically useless.

The oil of *H.venenata* or False Chaulmoogra (not found in Ceylon) has been examined by Brill (Phillipine Journ. of Sc. 1916, *11* [A], 75). It has been found that the chemical composition and constants are similar to those of *H. Wightiana*, *H.anthelmintica* and *Taraktogenos Kurzii*.

A cyanogenetic glucoside, identical with that found in G. odorata, has been found in Pangium edule, a plant found in various parts of the Phillipine Islands. The quantity of oil in the dry kernels is 21% (Phil. Journ. of Sc. 1917, *12*, 37; Abst. 1917, 1, 719).

The work of Power and his collaborators shows that true Chaulmoogra Oil is derived from the seeds of *Taraktogenos Kurzii* and that the oils from the two closely allied species of *Hydnocarpus* are practically identical. The oil from *G.odorata* is wholly different. It has been further shown by them that a new type of fatty acid is present in *Taraktogenos* and *Hydnocarpus* oils. These acids are strongly dextro-rotatory and contain a five-membered carbon ring with side-chains of different lengths. Brill, working on Phillipine plants, has confirmed the results of Power and has at the same time extended our knowledge of the distribution of the fatty acids in several species of plants related to those investigated by Power (vide, Brill, Phil. Journ. of Sc. Sec. A., 1916. *11*, 75; 1917, *12*, 37 & 207).

	H. Wightiana	H. anthelmintica	H. Venenata	H. alcalae	T. Kurzii	Pangium edule
M. P.	22°	24°	20°	32°	22°	Cloudy at 2°
Sp. Gr.	0.958 at 25°	0.953 at 25°	0.948 at 30°	0.950 at 30°	0.951 at 24°	0.905
Specific Rotation	+57.7	+52.5	+52.03	+49.6	+52	+4.28
Iodine Value	101.3	86.4	99.1	93.1	103.2	113.1
Chaulmoogric acid	+	+	+	90%	+	?
Hydnocarpic acid	+	+	+	—	+	?

Dean and Wrenshall (J. Am. Chem. Soc. 1920, *42*, 2626 give an account of the earlier work on the subject and their own results on the fractionation of the acids of chaulmoogra oil by fractional crystallisation of the acids and fractional distillation in high vacuum of the ethyl esters and the acids themselves. They find that there is no acid below hydnocarpic nor above chaulmoogric acid in the mixture. They also give a method for the nearly quantitative extraction of chaulmoogric and hydnocarpic acids from chaulmoogra oil.

Perkin and Cruz (Phil. Journ. of Sc., 1923, 23, 543) Abst. 1924, i, 486) examined the oils from the seeds of *G. odorata, H. alcalae, H. anthelmintica, H. Hitchinsonii, H.subfalcata, H.venenata, H.Wightiana, H.Woodii, Pangium edule* and *Taraktogenos Kurzii* and found a close similarity between the true chaulmoogra oil (from T. Kurzii) and all the Hydnocarpus oils investigated. The oil from *H.alcalae* contains a high percentage of chaulmoogric acid but contains little, if any, hydnocarpic acid.

It has been found by Schoble (Phil. Journ. of Sc., 1924, 24, 23; Abst. 1924, I, 690) that out of a large number of vegetable oils examined, chaulmoogra and hydnocarpus oils inhibit the growth of acid-fast bacteria best.

The toxicity of chaulmoogra oil has been investigated by Read (J. Pharm. Exp. Ther., 1924, *24*, 221; Abst. 1924, 1, 1377). He finds that toxic doses of hydnocarpate (ethyl and glyceryl) cause haemolysis, renal irritation and fatty infiltration of the liver. Increased lymph flow follows intravenous injection of ethyl hydnocarpate.

Read has also investigated the influence of Chaulmoogra oil on Calcium metabolism and that of hydnocarpates on urinary nitrogen partition in the dog (J. Biol. Chem. 1924, *62*, 513, 541; Abst. 1925. I, 194). He observes that large doses given to rabbits and dogs increase the excretion of calcium and also the nitrogen output.

Nord and Schweitzer (Abst. 1925, i, 734) are of opinion that the physiological activity of chaulmoogra, margosa, and hydnocarpus oils is independent of the nature of the unsaturated carbocyclic residue present in the component acids.

Wrenshall and Dean (Abst. 1925, i, 1414) have isolated from chaulmoogra oil a small quantity of a highly unsaturated acid, iodine val. 168.3 (probably $C_{17}H_{29}$. CO_2H), catalytic hydrogenation of which gives dihydrochaulmoogric acid, m.p., 71°. Dihydrohydnocarpic acid melts at 63°.

Power and his collaborators had not been able to investigate the nature of the residue left on fractional (vacuum) distillation. Hashimoto (J. Am. Chem. Soc. 1925, 47, 2325) has carried out this distillation under 0.01-0.05mm. pressure. He has obtained in this way the ethyl of (1) taraktogenic acid $C_{36}H_{60}O_6$, m.p. 113.5°; (2) isogadoleic acid $C_{20}H_{38}O_2$, m.p. 66°; (3) a lactone-like substance $C_{18}H_{32}O_2$, m.p. −11.6° etc. (vide also correction, J. Am. Chem. Soc. 1927, *49*, 1119).

The constitution of chaulmoogra and hydnocarpic acids have been worked out by Shriner and Adams who suggest that the former acid is l–(α –carboxy-*n*-dodecyl)–Δ^4–cyclopentene and the latter - l–(α –carboxy-*n*-dodecyl)–Δ^4–cyclopentene

$$\begin{array}{l} CH{=}CH \\ \vert \qquad\quad >CH\,(CH_2)_{12}\,CO_2H \text{ and} \\ CH_2{-}CH_2 \end{array}$$

$$\begin{array}{l} CH{=}CH \\ \vert \qquad\quad >CH\,(CH_2)_{10}CO_2H \text{ respectively} \\ CH_2{-}CH_2 \end{array}$$

For constitution see also Perkins, (J. Am. Chem. Soc. 1926, 48, 1714); van Dyke and Adams, (ibid, 2393;) Noller and Adams, (ibid, 2444.)

H. anthelmintica seeds from Ceylon examined at the Imperial Institute (Bull. Imp. Inst., 1929, 28,6) gave nearly the same results as those obtained by Power and Barrowcliff (J. Chem. Soc. 1905, 87, 89). The constituents of the oil were studied by the method of Perkin and Cruz (Phil. Journ. of Sc. 1923, 23, 557). Hydnocarpic and chaulmoogric acids were isolated.

BERBERIDEAE

Berberis aristata & Berberis asiatica, Eng. *Indian Barberry, Tree Turmeric;* Sinh. *Rasadun;* Sans. *Daruharidra, Pitadaru;* Tam. *Kasturi manjal, Maramanjal*, are erect much-branched bushes, having bright yellow flowers. *B.aristata, B. Lycium B.vulgaris* and *B.asiatica* are difficult to distinguish.

A crude extract known as *Rasaut, Rasavanti*, or *Rasanjana* is prepared from the root-bark for use as a local application in affections of the eyelids and in chronic opthalmia in which it is painted over the eyelids, occasionally combined with opium, rock-salt and alum. Its extracts are regarded as alterative and deobstruent and are given in jaundice and in affections of the eyes. Its tincture is used in cases of remittent and intermittent fevers and is very valuable in periodic neuralgia. As a diaphoretic and antipyretic it is said to be equal to quinine. Repeated doses of it do not produce cardiac depression or deafness, an advantage over quinine. It is given with butter in haemorrhoids. The root itself of *B.aristata* is found to be equal if not superior to the root-bark. This root, some believe, is "one of the few really good medicines of India" (Watt's Dict. of Econ. Products, Vol. 1, page 443).

Chemical and pharmacological investigations of several species of *Berberidiae* have been made. The first on record in the chemical literature is the examination of the berries of *B.vulgaris*, the species used in medicine in Europe, by Leńssen (Ber. 1870, *3*, 966). He found a very high content of free acid and a relatively low content of pectin bodies. Hesse (Ber. 1886, *19*, 3190) reinvestigated the alkaloids of *B.vulgaris*. He believed that there were four alkaloid bodies and described in particular two of them:—oxyacanthine, $C_{18}H_{19}O_3N$ and berbamine $C_{18}H_{19}O_3N.2H_2O$ from the mother liquors of the former. Oxyacanthine when crystallised from water and dried at 100° melts at 138-150°, but crystals from alcohol or ether melt at 208-214°. Berbamine crystallises in small scales of the composition $C_{18}H_{19}O_3N.2H_2O$. When anhydrous it melts at 156°

B. aquifolium, the species used in the United States and *B. vulgaris* have been investigated by Rudel (Arch. Pharm. 229, 631; Abst. 1892, i, 641). He assigns the formula $C_{19}H_{21}O_3N$ to oxyacanthine and finds that the substance melts between 174 and 185°. Berbamine $C_{18}H_{19}O_3N$ was separated by the addition of sodium nitrate and purified by precipitating the solution of the sulphate with ammonia and crystallizing from dry ether. His method consists in extracting the ground roots with acetic acid, precipitating oxyacanthine by the addition of sodium sulphate, berebine as acetone berberine and berbamine by the addition of sodium nitrate. All these three alkaloids are found in both the species. Poomerehne (Arch. Pharm. 1895, *233*, 127) confirms

Rudel's formula for oxyacanthine obtained from *B. aquifolium*. The substance is a mono-acid tertiary base. Berbamine appears to contain 1 or 2 methoxy groups.

From *B. Oetnensis* from Cyprus, Perkin (J. Chem. Soc. 1897, 71, 1198) isolated berberine as platinichloride and examined the nature of the dye, for which he found the plant useless.

Berberine is not toxic, in the ordinary sense, to the larger animals and man. In rabbits it produces respiratory disturbance and paresis.

GUTTIFERAE

Calophyllum Inophyllum,—Sinh. *Domba;* Sans. *Punnaga, Kesava;* Tam. *Punnaigam;* Eng. *Pannay tree, Alexandrian Laurel.*

This is a moderate-sized tree with a thick trunk and smooth grey bark and is common in the low country of Ceylon, principally the sea-coast. It grows throughout India.

The bark is used in decoction in internal haemorrhage. The leaves soaked in water are applied to inflamed eyes. An application for sore eyes is the oil obtained by steeping in water a mixture of the gum with strips of bark and leaves. The gum is also a remedy for wounds and ulcers. The seeds yield the well-known Domba Oil (called Laurel nut oil in India) which is used by the poorer classes for burning, and in medicine is highly esteemed as an external application in gonorrhoea, gleet and scabies and also used in hoof disease of cattle.

The Pharmacographia Indica states that the fresh kernels give off 39% water and that the dried kernels yield 68% of a greenish yellow, bitter and fragrant oil of specific gravity 0.9315 at 15°; it congeals at 19° and sets at 16°; saponification value 285.6. Fendler (Abst. 1905, ii, 277) made a chemical examination of the oil and found that the seeds contain 23-32% water and 51-55% oil which has a yellowish-green colour, a peculiar odour and a bitter taste. On standing it deposits fatty glycerides. It solidifies at 3°, melts again at 8° and has the following constants :—Sp. gr. 0.9428 at 15°; Reichert-Meissl value 0.13, Saponification value 196.0, acid value 28.4, iodine value 92.8, unsaponifiable matter 0.25%. Treatment with five per cent sodium hydroxide solution removes resinous matter. The oil purified in this way solidifies at 4°, melts again at 8° and has Reichert-Meissl value 0.18, saponification value 191 and iodine value 86. The fatty acids of the oil are chiefly palmitic, stearic and oleic.

Domba Oil is one of the "Five Oils" (*Pas-tel*) of the Sinhalese.

Calophyllum tomentosum, Eng. *Poon Spar, Sirpon Tree;* Sinh. *Keena;* Tam. *Pongu.*

A tall handsome tree with straight trunk and quadrangular twigs; it is a native of the moist low country of Ceylon, Western India and Malaya. The seeds yield an orange coloured oil (*keena-tel*) used in skin diseases and for lighting and other domestic purposes. The tree yields a black opaque gum which is very soluble in cold water and is feebly astringent. If the gum is steeped in water for some time, the solution becomes very dark in colour. Alum followed by sodium carbonate throws down some of the brown colouring matter without interfering with the fluorescence; in fact, after precipitation the solution is very strongly fluorescent. The solution gives an absorption band at the violet end of the spectrum but it is optically inactive. (Pharmacographia Ind.)

The variety growing on higher elevations is more striking and is *C. Walkerii.*

C. spectabile, Sinh. *Domba-keena;* Sans. *Sura Punnaga or Champayah* and *C. bracteatum* (Sinh. *Walu-keena*) have nearly the same properties as *Mesua ferrea.*

Garcinia Cambogia, Eng. *Red Mango,* Sinh. *Goraka;* Sans. *Tamala;* Tam. *Korakapuli.*

A moderate sized handsome tree with a round head and drooping branches and is a native of the moist low country of Ceylon and Western India. The large roundish fruit is of the size of an orange but has several vertical grooves. When ripe it is collected and the thick succulent shell is cut into sections, dried in the sun and preserved for use in the preparation of curries (as a substitute for the lime fruit) and also largely in the salting of fish.

The yellow resin, though not used in medicine, is purgative in action. It is made into a pigment by some Hindus to make sectarial marks. It is valueless as a pigment on account of its insolubility in water. It is, however, easily soluble in spirits of turpentine and may prove useful as a varnish.

Garcinia Morella, Sinh. *Gokatu,*— yields " Indian Gamboge," generally in the form of " tears " or "grains." Gamboge of commerce comes from Siam from *Garcinia Hanburyi.* The tree (which is of slow growth and for tapping must not be less than 12 years old) is tapped during the rainy season, a spiral groove being cut round the trunk. The yellowish viscous liquid trickles along the cut and is collected into small bamboos placed below. The Gamboge of *G. Morella* is little collected in Ceylon but in Burma it is used as a yellow dye for the silk robes of Buddhist monks.

A semi-solid fat of a yellow colour is obtained in moderate yield from the seeds. It is employed as a lamp-oil and may prove useful for the manufacture of candles.

Garcinia mangostana, Eng. *Mangosteen.*

It is not used medicinally. It was introduced into Ceylon about 1800 from Malaya. The fruit is delicious and is in season in the low country of Ceylon from May to July and at higher elevations from July to August or September to October.

By boiling the rind of the fruit, first with water and then with alcohol, and allowing the alcoholic solution to stand, Schmid (Ann. 1855, 93, 83) obtained a substance, which he named mangostin. Liechti prepared the same substance in bright yellow, slender laminae, m. p., 173° and assigned to it the formula $C_{20}H_{22}O_5$.

Garcinia echinocarpa, Sinh. *Madol,*— is a tall tree of the Central and Southern Provinces of Ceylon. The seeds yield a thick oil used for burning and said to be used in medicine. As a lamp oil it is of indifferent value.

Mesua ferrea, Eng. *Ceylon Iron Wood tree,* Sinh. *Na;* Sans. *Nagakesara;* Tam. *Nagacuram.*

A slow growing tree having crimson coloured leaves when tender, and delicately scented white flowers with yellow centre of numerous stamens.

The leaves are used in the form of poultice which is applied to the head in severe colds. A paste of the flowers is applied to bleeding piles and for burning of the feet. A syrup of the flower buds is given in dysentery.

The seeds yield a thick, dark coloured oil which is used as an application for sores, scabies, etc., and is also used as an embrocation in rheumatism. When extracted with ether the seeds yield 31.5% of fixed oil, of a deep yellow colour, sp. gr. 0.972 at 17° at which temperature the oil sets.

An oleo-resin abounds in all parts of the tree and is obtained pure from the young fruits. It melts at 50-60°, is entirely soluble in benzene but only partially in alcohol and ether. With ammonia it forms a clear mixture which gives a curdy precipitate on the addition of acid. The solution in alcohol is acid in reaction and is dextro-rotatory. On distillation it gives 0.6% of a fragrant essential oil, having the same smell as the flowers.

DIPTEROCARPACEAE

These are trees with resinous wood, many species of which are found in Ceylon. Only a few of them, however, are used in medicine.

Dipterocarpus glandulosus, Sinh. *Dorana;* Sans. *Guga;* Tam. *Yennai,*—is a tall erect tree from the stem of which exudes naturally a resin which may be collected at the base. This is used as a furniture varnish and for mixing paints. In medicine it is applied externally to rheumatic swellings and chronic inflammatory enlargements.

Dipterocarpus turbinatus, is the Garjan oil tree or Wood Oil tree of India; it yields the "Garjan" balsam of commerce. It has been used, but without much success, in the treatment of leprosy.

Dipterocarpus Zeylanicus, Sinh. *Hora,*—is a timber tree but the heart-wood is sometimes used as an ingredient in decoctions for fever. Klimont (Abst. 1905, ii, 126) has examined a sample of tallow (from Borneo) from the fruits of this species and obtained the following values: m. p. 34.5°, acid value 15.8, iodine value 30.1, saponification value 194.6 and that it contains tristearin, tripalmitin (?), oleodistearin and oleodipalmitin.

Gurjun Balsam Oil, erroneously known as East Indian Copaiba Balsam is designated "wood oil" in India, where considerable amounts of it are used as varnish. It is obtained from a variety of species of *Dipterocarpus.* In British East India two kinds of related balsams are differentiated: Kanyin oil, which presumably is the true balsam and "In" oil. These two oils differ appreciably both as to physical and chemical properties. The difference is partly due to the method of production: kanyin oils are produced with the aid of heat and the "In" oils without.

A sample from *D. turbinatus* examined was a slightly acid (acid value 10.9), milky liquid of specific gravity 0.9811 at 15°. Upon standing in a warm place, it separated into a brown oil and a tough greyish white emulsion-like mass. The oily layer gave the following values :—Sp. gr. at 15°0. 9706, $[\alpha]_D - 10°8'$, $n^{20°}_D$ 1.5120, acid value 7.3, E. V. 1.9.

" In " oil from Borneo gave sp. gr. 1.029, acid value 17.8, E. V. 0. (from Gildemeister and Hoffmann's Volatile Oils, iii, 173.)

Dryobalanops aromatica, Eng. *Borneo or Sumatra Camphor,* Sinh. *Gaskapuru;* Sans. *Karpura;* Tam. *Kapuran-shudan.*

A large forest tree which yields a camphor-like resin used in Chinese medicine. In the crevices and cracks of the trunks of older trees the highly-prized Borneo Camphor is found. The Malays, who designate the resin Kayu Kapur, use it for embalming the dead and for other ritual. In addition to this camphor, the tree yields a volatile oil obtained either by tapping the trees or by the distillation of the wood. Some trees contain solid borneol, others only a volatile oil because, (in Janse's opinion), of the presence of the larvae of beetles (probably), which bore through the wood ; in these passages the volatile oil collects.

Schimmel & Co's examination of a sample of the oil from Singapore gave the following results :—colour, dark-brown ; sp. gravity at 15°, 0.9180 ; $[\alpha]_D + 11°5'$ n_D 1.4885.

For an account of the composition, etc. of the volatile oil, (See Gildemeister & Hoffmann, iii, 168.)

Vateria acuminata, Sinh. *Hal;* Sans. *Aswakarna;* Tam. *Kungiliyam,*—is a large, handsome, upright tree, with spreading branches and a round head. Its fruit is large and pear-shaped. It is peculiar to the moist low country of Ceylon up to 2,000 feet.

The tree yields a clear, yellowish resin (considered equal to the best dammar), which exudes abundantly from the stem. This resin is astringent and emolient and is used in dysentery. Like other gums it is used as a fumigator for sick rooms. The bark is astringent and bitter and is used in medicine in conjunction with other drugs. It is commonly used for retarding the fermentation of toddy. In Ceylon, when *Hal* bark is not available, fermentation is checked by lining the inside of the container.

Vateria indica var malabarica, Tam. *Vellai-kungiliyam, Pinaimaṛam, Dhupmaram.*

This tree is indigenous to S. W India, Canara and Travancore. It yields a true resin of considerable value known as White Dammar or Piney Resin. It occurs (according to Watt) in three forms :—First, Compact Piney Resin, in lumps of all shapes, varies in colour, on the outside from bright orange to dull yellow has a bright vitreous fracture, and internally presents all shades of colour from a light green to a light yellow. It bears a general resemblance to amber and may be easily distinguished from all other Indian resins. Second, Cellular Piney Resin occurs either in small lumps or in large masses, generally of a shining appearance and balsamic smell. It has a distinctly cellular structure, partly owing to the method of collection and partly to the age of the tree. Notches are cut in the trunk of the tree sloping downwards and inwards, the resin collects in the cavity and is either permitted to dry *in situ* or is collected and dried by heat. Third, dark-coloured Piney Resin is occasionally obtained on splitting open old and decayed trees. It has the solid consistence of the first, but the inferior quality of the second variety. (Watt's Dictionary of Econ. Products.)

In most of the properties Piney Resin resembles copal but it also possesses certain superior qualities. Like copal, it is only slightly soluble in spirit but dissolves readily on the addition of a little camphor to the spirit. Its solution in chloroform might be used as a substitute for amber in photographer's varnish. It is superior to copal in that it is soluble in turpentine and drying oils without the necessity of the preliminary destructive fusion required by that resin—a process which impairs the colour of the varnish.

Watt gives the following recipe for the preparation of a varnish. Into a new and perfectly clean earthen vessel put one part of Piney Dammar in coarse powder, cover closely and apply a very gentle heat, until the whole is melted; then add about two parts of linseed oil nearly boiling hot and mix well with a wooden spatula. Should the varnish prove too thick, it can, at any time, be reduced by the addition of more oil, or, if required may be made thicker in the first instance. Close covering, complete liquefaction of the resin, and boiling hot oil are absolutely necessary to the success of the process.

Vateria malabarica has been investigated chemically. The fatty matter is known as Piney or Malabar Tallow. Two samples of this vegetable tallow, one obtained from Venice and the other from Trieste were examined by dal Sie (Abst. 1878, 764). He found that it contained free palmitic acid 75% and free oleic acid 22.8%, besides a small quantity of impurity. The presence of volatile matter or glycerol could not be detected. The crude fat after filtration was bleached by mixing it with an equal bulk of boiling water, adding 9% of nitric acid and boiling for a few minutes: the original greenish colour changes to yellow and a subsequent exposure to the sun and air, after the acid has been removed by washing with boiling water, easily completes the bleaching process. In this form it makes good candles.

Hohnel and Wolfbauer (Abst. 1886, 223) note that the tallow is rapidly bleached on exposure to light. It is rapidly saponified yielding a mixture of fatty acids melting at 56.6° and resolidifying at 54.8°, and consisting of oleic acid and some solid fatty acids melting at 63.8°.

The following are the characteristics of Malabar Tallow: Sp. gr. 0.9102 at 9.4° (dal Sie), 0.915 at 15° (H & W), 0.8907 at 100° (Crossley & Le Sueur); Solidifying point 30.5°; m. p. 36.5°, 30° (dal Sie). 42° (H & W), 37.5° (C & Le Sueur); Sap. Val. 189-192; Iod. Val. 37.8- 29.6.

MALVACEAE

Abutilon indicum and asiaticum, Eng. *Country mallow*, Sinh. *Anoda*; Sans. *Atibala, Kangkatika* (Atygalle gives *Kalikanghi* and *Balbija*); Tam. *Peruntutti.*

Abutilon asiaticum is rather rare and grows on waste ground, chiefly in the low country; *Abutilon indicum* is common in the dry country. The former flowers in July to September (yellow) and the latter most of the year (orange-yellow).

The leaves are smashed and boiled with rice flour for use as a poultice for sores, which is as good as linseed meal for the purpose. An infusion of the leaves or of the roots is given in fevers. The flowers and leaves are used as a local application for boils and ulcers. The decoction of the leaves is used also as a fomentation to painful parts. The seeds are considered laxative and demulcent and given in fevers as a cooling remedy. They are used in decoction in haemorrhoids and are also said to be useful in gonorrhoea, gleet and chronic cystitis. They are also said to be useful in the treatment of leprosy. The bark and root are diuretic.

The leaves are said to contain mucilage, tannin, organic acids and traces of asparagin. (Pharm. Ind.)

A fibre can be obtained from this genus and ought to be investigated.

Adansonia digitata, Eng. *Baobab Tree,* Tam. *Anai-puli-maram.*

This is a low tree of great girth and is a native of Central Africa. It is famous for the great girth and age to which it attains. A few trees have long been established in Mannar (Ceylon) whither it was brought long ago by Arab traders. The largest tree found there in 1890 was, according to Crawford, 61 feet in girth and 30 feet in height. The Tamils call it *Papparappuli* or *Anaipuliya-maram* and the Roman Catholics call it *Judas' Bag*. The Sanskrit name is *Gorak-amli,* obviously a recent name. It is supposed to be one of the longest lived trees. The wood is soft and spongy and the inner bark fibrous. The white gourd-like fruits are spongy, acid and edible. Slocum (Abst. 1880, 836) has found in the fruit pectin, glucose and malic acid but not a trace of tartaric acid.

The fibre from the inner bark is used for ropes and cordage in Madagascar and Africa.

The bark when wounded yields a large quantity of white semi-fluid gum which is inodorous and tasteless. The ash contains a large quantity of lime. Gum Baobab is insoluble in water and appears to be allied to Gum Tragacanth.

Bombax malabaricum, Eng. *Red Silk Cotton Tree,* Sinh. *Katu-imbul ;* Sans. *Raktashalmali, Maha-vriksha, Pancha-parni ;* Tam. *Parutti.*

A very large, handsome, upright, quick-growing deciduous tree, reaching a height of 120 feet or more and is a native of Ceylon, India, Burma, etc. Its flowers are large, fleshy and bright red. When the tree flowers, usually in January and February, it is leafless and presents a very striking sight. The trunk is used for making canoes.

The bark is astringent and is used in the form of a paste externally in inflammations and cutaneous eruptions. The gum exuding from the tree is demulcent and astringent; it is called *Mocharas* in Sanskrit and *Himbul* or *Imbul-latu* in Sinhalese. It is largely used in cases of dysentery, diarrhoea, menorrhagia and other affections in which astringents like *kino* and *catechu* are useful.

The following is a very well-known prescription in dysentery of children: Gum of *Bombax malabaricum Mimosa pudica, Woodfordia floribunda* and stamens of *Nymphaea* (lotus,) in decoction prepared in the usual way. The petals squeezed and soaked in milk form a soothing application for conjunctivitis of infants. The dry young fruits are beneficial in calculous affections and chronic inflammation and ulceration of the bladder and kidneys.

The seeds are said to have good effects in gonorrhoea. The "cotton" is employed externally on account of its softness and elasticity in padding splints and covering burnt and inflamed surfaces.

Eriodendron anfractuosum, Eng. *Kapok-tree, white silk cotton tree*, Sans. *Salmali*; Sinh. *Imbul, Pulun*; Tam. *Illanku.*

This is a small or moderate-sized, quick-growing, upright tree, branching horizontally. It is deciduous in the dry season, usually February to April. The fruit pods which open about two months after flowering contain a quantity of silky, creamy white floss (Kapok), consisting of unicellular hairs. This kapok is used for stuffing pillows, etc., and, mixed with other fibres, for weaving into fine fabrics.

The medicinal properties and uses are the same as those of *B. malabaricum.*

Lewkowitsch (ii, 185) gives an account of "kapok" oil which he describes as the oil from the seeds of *Eriodendron anfractuosum* and *Bombax malabaricum,* but does not distinguish between the individual oils from the two sources.

The seeds contain 24.2% oil and 15.9% carbohydrates. The oil has a greenish-yellow colour and a not unpleasant taste and odour. The following are the constants: Sp. gr. at 18°, 0. 9199; Sap. Val. 181-205; Iod. Val. 118-129 or 85.24 - 93.78. Like cotton-seed oil, it deposits stearine on standing, and has similar colour reactions. The acids are mainly palmitic and stearic. In Europe it is used in soap-making.

Reinders (Abst. 1877, i, 105) has examined the manurial value of Kapok cake and found 26.34% of nitrogenous compounds as against 20.62% in cotton-seed oil.

Details of cultivation, etc. are given in The Bull. of the Imp. Inst., 1911, page 121.

Gossypium Stocksii var herbaceum, Eng. *cotton,* Sinh. *Kapu,*—thrives in Ceylon in the dry regions of the Northern, North-Central and Southern Provinces. The seeds are frequently used in the treatment of urinary diseases. A poultice made of cotton seed, ginger and water is applied in orchitis. The seed is largely used in feeding milch cows. Its general properties and uses are similar to those of Kapok.

For the chemistry, etc. of cotton seed oil, see Lewkowitsch, ii, 187.

Hibiscus Abelmoschus, Linn., Eng. *The Musk Mallow,* Sinh. *Kapukinissa;* Sans. *Latakasturika;* Tam. *Vattilai-kasturi, Katukasturi.*

A herbaceous bush common throughout the hotter parts of India.

The seeds (known in European trade as grains of Ambrette) give an odorous principle employed as a substitute for musk. In medicine they are useful in nervous debility, hysteria and other nervous diseases, in atonic dyspepsia and in a few other conditions in which the use of musk is indicated. They are also used in perfuming medicinal oils. Powdered seeds steeped in alcohol are applied to the bites of snakes. The root and leaves are recommended in gonorrhoea. No part of the plant is, however, recognized as of value by the Pharmacopoeia of India.

The stems yield a fibre, the strength of which does not appreciably diminish with wetting.

The fixed oil from the seeds is a greenish yellow liquid, fluid at 0°, but solidifies gradually on exposure to the air. The solid crystalline matter was deposited from the hot alcoholic solution of the seeds ; it was white, pearly, of a pleasant taste, soluble in ether from which it crystallises in rays fusible at 35°.

Gildermeister and Hoffmann (iii, 160) give an account of the essential oil obtained from the seeds. It was first prepared by Schimmel & Co. in 1887, obtaining a yield of 0.2 - 0.6%. It is a "concrete" mass, resembling orris oil. Liquid ambrette seed oil introduced into commerce by Schimmel & Co. in 1902 is free from the inodorous (hence valueless and for the most part objectionable) fatty acid. Constants :—$D_{15°}$ 0.905 to 0.917 ; $[\alpha]_D$ slightly dextrogyrate up to 1° 20′, rarely laevogyrate up to −2° 24′; $n_D^{20°}$ 1.474 - 1.480; E. V. 137-190.

Farnesol, $C_{15}H_{24}O$, is the only known constituent of ambrette seed oil. In the aqueous distillate furfural has been found. The bulk of the ordinary ambrette seed oil is palmitic acid.

Hibiscus esculentus Linn, Eng. "*Lady's Fingers*" *or Ochru* (*West Indies*); Sinh. *Bandakka;* Sans. *Tindisha;* Tam. *Vendaikkai.*

It is an erect annual, bearing erect horn-like pods. When immature it forms an agreeable, mucilaginous vegetable. It is not used in medicine in Ceylon, but in India the mucilage of the fruit and seeds is used as demulcent in gonorrhoea and in irritation of the genito-urinary system.

Zega's analysis (Abst. 1901, ii, 70) of a Servian specimen shows the following percentage composition ;—water 80.74, nitrogenous material 4.15, fat 0.42, carbohydrates 12.12, etc.

Roxburgh mentions that the stigmas are replete with a very beautiful, deep-purple juice which they communicate to paper and which is tolerably durable. Murray in his "Plants and Drugs of Sind" confirms this and adds that the stained paper forms a substitute for litmus paper. The writer can find no further record of the employment of the colouring matter as a dye.

The bast yields a strong useful fibre of a white colour, which is long and silky, generally, strong and pliant. It is employed economically in some parts of India, but in many districts where the plant is much grown as a vegetable the excellence of the fibre seems to be unrecognized. It is undoubtedly valuable and seems to possess qualities specially fitting it for the purposes of paper-making. (Watt.)

Hibiscus rosa-sinensis, Eng. Shoe-flower Sinh. *Wadamal Sapattumal;* Sans. *Jova, Rudra-pushpa; Japa-pushpa.* Tam. *Shappattuppu.;*

A tall shrub occurring in many varieties. It is a native of China but is found in the plains of India.

The flowers are astringent and are used in uterine haemorrhage. They are also refrigerant, emollient, demulcent and aphrodisiac. They are fried with ghee and given in menorrhagia. The buds are employed in the cure of seminal weakness. The root is valuable in cough. A stimulating application for the hair is made by mixing the juice of the fresh petals and olive oil in equal portions and boiling it till all the water has evaporated.

Hibiscus sabdariffa, Linn., Eng. *Rozelle or Red Sorrel* (of West Indies) is cultivated in gardens and occasionally occurs wild. It has no Sinhalese name and is apparently not used by the Sinhalese medical men. It is grown as a food-plant in India in the North-West Provinces and the Punjab. The stems yield the Rozelle hemp of commerce which is obtained by retting the twigs as soon as the plant is in flower. The red calyces are employed for dyeing. Perkin (J. Chem. Soc. 1909, 95, 1855) has examined the colouring matters of the flowers, etc. (It should be noted, however, that the material used by Perkin had considerably deteriorated during transport). According to him the colouring matter is Gossypetin, the colouring matter of the flowers of the Indian cotton plant. (Vide J. Chem. Soc. 1899, 75, 825). In the former paper Perkin revises the formula of gossypetin to $C_{15}H_{10}O_8$. It gives a hexa-acetyl derivative. He also isolated protocatechuic acid, crystallising from water and melting at 194-196°, which, however, is, in his opinion a decomposition product, and a pale yellow substance melting at about 340° (with decomposition) giving a sparingly soluble acetyl derivative, m.p. 239°. This substance, for which the name Hibiscetin is proposed, dyes mordanted calico.

Hibiscus cannabinus, Linn., Deccan or Bombay or Ambar-Hemp—is found near cooly lines on Ceylon plantations or as an occasional weed but is not native nor is it much cultivated. It is a small herbaceous plant cultivated in India and Africa for the fibre obtained from the inner bark. It is very much superior to jute. In India a coarse sack-cloth is made from it though its chief use is for ropes and cordage.

Hibiscus tiliaceus, Linn., Sinh. *Bellipatta,*—is a small tree or bush thriving near rivers. It yields a fibre of fair quality which can be readily separated and does not easily rot under water. In Ceylon it is used for making ropes and mats. The root is employed in India as a febrifuge and in the preparation of an embrocation. It is not used medicinally in Ceylon.

Pavonia odorata, Willd. Sinh. *Pushpa-bevila;* Sans. *Bala, Hrivera;* Tam. *Paramutiver.*

An erect branched annual herb. *Pavonia zeylanica* is a much branched perennial herb. These herbs and their roots have a musklike odour. The roots are regarded as cooling, demulcent, carminative, diaphoretic and diuretic and are largely used in combination with other drugs for fever and affections of the chest. They are also useful in haemorrhage from internal organs. *P.odotara* is an ingredient in the drink (for fever) " Shadanga Paniya."

The therapeutic properties of the root are probably due to the carminative quality of the odorous matter it contains, together with the mucilaginous character commonly met with in members of the *Malvaceae.*

Both species yield a fibre of excellent quality, which somewhat resembles that obtained from the fibre-yielding species of *Hibiscus.* It is of a finer texture, softer and whiter, with a cellulose content of 74.7%.

Sida humilis, Willd. Sinh. *Bevila;* Tam. *Palampadu.*
Sida mysorensis. Sinh. *Siriwadi-bevila.*
Sida acuta. Sinh. *Gas-bevila.*
Sida rhombifolia. (Roxb.) Sinh. *Kotikan-bevila;* Tam. *Chittamaddi.*
Sida cordifolia, Linn. Sinh. *Wal-bevila or Heen-anoda;* Tam. *Chevakanpudu.*

These are perennial herbs used in Sinhalese medicine indiscriminately, with the same effect, one for another for the five kinds of "bala" of the Sanskrit writers. *Bevila* is considered cooling, astringent and tonic and is given in fever and urinary complaints. Singly or in combination with other drugs it is given to women during the whole period of gestation, sometimes as a preventive of miscarriages and abortion. The powder of the root-bark is useful in frequent micturition, leucorrhoea and gonorrhoea.

S. rhomboidea, of which *S. rhombifolia* is a variety, yields a fibre which has a relatively high percentage of cellulose, 83.0% whereas jute contains only 75%.

Thespesia populnea, Corr., "*Tulip tree*", Sinh. *Sooriya;* Sans. *Parisa;* Tam. *Kavarachu, Puvarachu.*

It is a small much-branched spreading tree. Its heartwood is used for making furniture. It is not much used in medicine in Ceylon; the decoction of the bark is, however, given as an astringent, tonic and alterative.

Thespesia lampas is a small bush common to the tropical jungles of India, Burma and Ceylon. Perkin (J. Chem. Soc. 1909, 95, 1859) has investigated the colouring matter of the yellow sepals of this plant. 250 grams of the material gave 1.5 grams of the crude dye, which is a glucoside crystallising from dilute alcohol in colourless needles, m. p. 191-194°. The compound possessed all the properties of acetyl-quercetin and gave carbon and hydrogen combustion values agreeing with $C_{15}H_5O_7 (C_2H_3O)_5$. The aqueous filtrate contained protocatechuic acid as in *Hibiscus sabdariffa.* The amount of material available for this research was small.

Wisadula zeylanica, Medik. Sinh. *Wisadooliya, Kirikaju;* Sans. & Tam. *Wisadooliya.*

An erect shrubby plant, 5-6 feet high, common in the low country of Ceylon and Tropics generally. Its stem gives a good fibre.

As its Sinhalese name implies, it is an antidote to snake poison. The plant has not been scientifically investigated.

STERCULIACEAE

Helicteres Isora, Linn., Eng. *East Indian Screw Tree;* Sinh. *Leeniya;* Sans. *Mrigashenga (deer's horn), Avatarni;* Tam. *Valumbirikai.*

A shrub or small tree, with hazel-like leaves, common in Tropical Asia, and in Ceylon in the low country. The inner bark gives a very tough fibre.

The capsule, which consists of five linear, many-sided carpels, spirally twisted, and terminating in a thick point to form a cone, has long been employed medicinally in India. Its use, however, seems to depend almost entirely on the ancient Doctrine of Signatures, the peculiarly twisted carpels being supposed to resemble the folds of the intestines. (Pharm. Ind.) The fruits are thus employed in intestinal disturbances such as colic. It is also given to relieve gripe and flatulence in children. In some parts of India, the root bark is used in diabetes and is said to lessen the quantity of sugar in the urine.

The fibre from the bast resembles jute in appearance and contains 56% of cellulose.

Pentapetes Phoenicea, Linn., Sinh. *Banduwada;* Sans. *Bandhu. ka, Bandhujeeva, Raktaka, Arkavallaba, Pushparakta;* Tam- *Nagapu.*

A slightly branched annual with bright-red flowers. It is very rare in Ceylon, and is found in the dry parts. There are three other varieties in India. The fruit is used medicinally with other drugs, on account of its mucilaginous properties, for diseases of the bowels.

Pterospermum suberifolium, Linn. Sinh. *Welanga;* Sans. *Moochukunda;* Tam. *Vinanku.*

A rather small tree growing in India and Burma and common in the dry regions of the low country of Ceylon.

The flowers are yellowish white and are very sweet-scented.

The flowers made into a paste with rice-vinegar or Kanjika form the ancient and well-known application for Hemicrania. No essential oil has yet been distilled from them.

Sterculia acerifolia, the Flame Tree of Queensland,—is a native of Australia, introduced to Ceylon in 1882. It is suited to higher altitudes and produces in May and June large masses of brilliant red blossoms.

Sterculia Balanghas, Linn., Sinh. *Nawa;* Tam. *Vellai Puttalai,*—is a tree with showy fruits, the bright orange carpels of which open exposing large jet-black shiny seeds. It is common in the low country of Ceylon and in India and Malaya. Its inner bark yields a fibre used in making ropes and hats.

Sterculia foetida, Linn. Sinh. *Telambu;* Eng. *Poon tree or Wild almond;* Sans. *Ashtakshara;* Tam. *Kudrapdukku.*

A large tree, common in the low country of Ceylon, especially the dry regions, and in India on the Western Ghats and Southern India. It is also widely distributed in the Dutch Indies, Indo-China, the East Indies and Malaya. It is cultivated for its wood, which in its green state has an unpleasant smell. The seeds are known in commerce as Olives of Java, *Kalvempang beans, Beligno seeds or Sterculia kernels.*

The leaves are considered as repellent and aperient. The seeds bring on nausea and vertigo.

The seeds examined at the Imperial Institute yielded 2.5% epicarp, 16% mesocarp, 33% shell and 48% kernel. The kernel contained 52.1% of oil, that is, 30.8% of the nut. The extracted kernel oil is liquid but slightly viscous, the expressed oil is somewhat insipid. The oil obtained from the whole seed by extraction or expression is liquid and slightly viscous. It has the same colour, taste and odour as the kernel oil but on standing stearine separates out at the ordinary temperature.

The most characteristic property of *Sterculia oil* is that on heating to 240-245°, it polymerises with spontaneous evolution of heat into an india-rubber like solid substance. If the oil is heated to 240° and the temperature not allowed to rise above 250°, a tough india-rubber-like mass is obtained which remains elastic on exposure to the air and is insoluble in the usual solvents. This phenomenon has not been thoroughly investigated.

The following are the constants of the oil :—

	Sp. gr.at 15°	Sap. Value	Iodine val.
Pulp oil	—	172.4 - 193.8	57 - 81
Kernel oil	0.929	192.5 - 212.0	81 - 87
Whole oil	0.9260	187.9	76.6

For details see Lewkowitsch, ii, 386 et seq.

The results of an examination of the Polymer are found in Lewkowitsch, iii, 141 :— Saponification value 184.9-184.5; Iodine value 76.0-76.3 unsaponifiable matter 1.16% Wedemeyer who discovered this polymerisation proposed the use of the substance as a substitute for rubber.

In medicine the chief use of the oil is as a fumigatory. In itch and other skin diseases it is given internally and the paste of the seeds applied externally. In India the oil is extracted by boiling with water. The bark and leaves are aperient, diuretic and diaphoretic.

Sterculia urens, Roxb.,—is "*Balika*" of the Sanskrit writers and "*Kavali*" of the Tamils ; its Sinhalese name has not been ascertained.

Sterculia acuminata, Eng. *Kola nut,*—is a native of West Africa, now cultivated in India but not in Ceylon. The nut is a valuable dietetic agent, sustaining the system against fatigue. Heckel and Schlagdenhauffen (Compt. rend., *94*. 802; Abst. 1882, 1125) have found the following constituents;—Substances soluble in chloroform, caffeine 2.348%, theobromine 0.023%, tannin 0.027%, fatty matters 0.585%; soluble in alcohol, tannin 1.591%, kola red 1.290%, glucose 2.875%, fixed salts 0.070%; other substances, starch 33.7%, gum, colouring matters, proteids, cellulose, etc.

Natton (J. Pharm. 5, *10*, 257; Abst. 1885, 712) remarks that the nut possesses tonic, nutritive, exciting and aphrodisiacal properties. It is employed either fresh or roasted. It is astringent and tonic and is recommended for chronic diarrhoea, cardiacal affections and cachexy.

The mucilage from the young shoots of *S.plantanifolia* (not found in Ceylon) contains arabans with some galactans. (Yoshimura, Abst. 1896, ii, 60)

TILIACEAE

Corchorus capsularis, Linn., and *C. olitorious,* Eng. *Jute or Gunny fibre;* Sinh. *Jaladara, wanuk;* Sans. *Nadika, Patta, Singikka;* Tam. *Piratti-kirai.*

These are annual plants, with long, erect, thin stem and yellow flowers. They are indigenous to many parts of India and to Ceylon.

The leaves are demulcent, bitter, tonic, stomachic laxative, carminative, refrigerant and diuretic. An infusion of the plant is used as a beverage in fevers. An infusion of the leaves with coriander is a domestic remedy for colic.

Jute is the bast fibre almost exclusively of these two plants. It is, as is well-known, very largely used for the manufacture of sacking and wrapping cloths (Hessians), as a paper-making fibre or as a substitute for hair in making theatrical wigs; also for carpet making and inferior cordage. According to the investigations of Cross and Beven jute does not contain cellulose as such, but as bastose or lignocellulose, which is a link between the carbohydrates and aromatic compounds. Treated with chlorine, it gives a yellow chlorinated derivative, which yields on hydrolysis substances belonging to the tannic acid group. When treated with acids, jute yields xylose and furfural.

Annett (Biochem. J., 1917, *11*, 1; Abst. 1917, i, 506) found that the seeds of the jute plant contain 2-3% of raffinose. A glucoside, corchorin, is present in the seeds of *C.capsularis*. Another glucoside, capsularin, has been isolated by Saha and Choudhury (J. Chem. Soc., 1922, *121*, 1044) from the leaves of the same plant, by extraction with water. The substance is very bitter to the taste and is sparingly soluble in water, insoluble in ether, but readily soluble in alcohol. It has been assigned the formula, $C_{22}H_{36}O_8$, and gives a penta-acetyl derivative. On hydrolysis it gives glucose and a substance crystallising from acetic acid and melting at 185°

Grewia tiliaefolia, Vahl. Sinh. *Hamaniya*; Sans. *Dharmana, Dhamni;* Tam. *Chaddchchi,*—is astringent and cooling and is prescribed in dysentery.

Grewia polygama, Roxb., Sinh. *Bora-damaniya;* Tam. *Taviddai,*—Its fruit is used by the Santals in cases of diarrhoea and dysentery, for which the powdered root is also used. The root, powdered in water, is applied externally to hasten suppuration and as dressing for wounds.

Grewia scabrophylla, Roxb.,—a species of *Damaniya*, is regarded as a remedy for leprosy, in accordance with the Doctrine of Signatures. It appears to be simply mucilaginous like most of the species. Its roots are used in Goa as a substitute for Althaea.

Grewia populifolia, Sinh. *Katuperatti;* Tam. *Achchu.* The pulp of the fruit is pleasantly acid.

RUTACEAE

Acronychia laurifolia, Sinh. *Ankenda.*

A small tree, with pale smooth bark and pale-yellow flowers. It is common and grows in moist regions up to 5000 feet ; it is also found in Bengal, South West India, Malaya and Cochin China. The whole plant when bruised has a warm terebinthanate scent. The bark is used as an external application to sores and ulcers (Trimen). The leaves give an oil, D_{26° 0.95, $[\alpha]_D 1^\circ 52'$, Sap. Value 11; it contained no aldehydes.

The following are said to be used in medicine :—

Evodia Roxburghiana, Sinh. *Lunu-ankenda,*—is a small tree, common in the moist country from 2000-6000 ft.

Evodia meliaefolia, is found in China and Japan, where its bark is employed in dyeing as well as in medicine. It is synonymous with *Evodia glauca* of India. The colouring matter of the bark has been investigated by Perkin and Hummel (J. Chem. Soc., 1895, 67, 414). They found berberine in it.

Glycosmis pentaphylla, Correa, Sinh. *Dodanpana;* Tam. *Kulapannai,*—is an evergreen shrub found throughout India and Ceylon. The roots powdered and mixed with sugar are given in cases of low fever.

Micromelum pubescens, Sinh. *Wal-karapincha;* Tam. *Kakaipalai,*—is a small tree rather common in the low country, especially in the dry regions. Its flowers are white and strong smelling. The scent of the leaves is fairly aromatic. It is easily confounded with *Murraya Koenigii* and *Clausena indica.*

Clausena indica, Oliv., Sinh. *Meegon-karapincha;* Tam. *Pannai, Purankainari,*—is a small tree or shrub, rather common in the low country, principally in the dry region. The leaves are fairly aromatic and the fruit edible.

Toddalia aculeata, Pers., Sinh. *Kudu-miris;* Sans. *Kanchana, Dahana;* Tam. *Milakaram, Kandai,*—is a small erect or climbing, prickly shrub and is very common. It appears to have been one of the plants known to Sanskrit writers as *Kanchana,* golden, on account of the orange colour of the fruit. Its other Sanskrit name *Dahana* is due to the pungency of its berries.

The fresh leaves are eaten raw for pains in the bowels. The ripe berries are as pungent as pepper. Roxburgh was of opinion that the herb might prove a valuable medicine where stimulants are required. The root, pounded with oil, is applied externally to rheumatic swellings. It is of great value in constitutional debility and in convalescence after exhausting diseases. In decoction, the root is given for intermittent fever. The berries are pickled.

The whole plant is bitter ; Perkin and Hummel (J. Chem. Soc., 1895, 67, 413) have found berberine in the bark but none in the wood. It was introduced into European medicine in 1771 as Lopez Root but has long since fallen into disuse.

The oil from the root bark contains a volatile oil, the odour of which is described as cinnamon and balm-like. " On distillation the leaves yield a pale yellowish green limpid oil, having the odour of citron peel, and a bitter and aromatic taste. The specific gravity at 17° is 0.873 ; examined by polarized light in a tube of 200 mm. it rotates 15°30' to the left. The oil has no constant boiling point, but the greater part distils over between 190° and 210°. Metallic sodium has a slight action upon it, which causes a yellow colour, and a white deposit in the oil." (Pharm. Ind.) D. Hopper (Schimmel's Reports, 1893,73) also distilled the oil and found considerable amounts of citronellal and an alcoholic constituent which boils above 200°. Brooks (Phillip. Journal Sc., 1911, *6A* 344) also examined the oil and obtained the following results :—Sp. gr. 0.9059, $n_D^{30°}$ 1.4620. On cooling 18% of a solid smelling like camphor but decomposing easily, separated ; Crystals from ligroin melted at 97° The 195-200° fraction contained linalool.

None of the constituents of the *Toddalia* root have been satisfactorily examined.

Aegle marmelos, Corr., Eng. *Bael fruit,* (slime apple) *Bengal Quince;* Sinh. *Beli;* Sans. *Vilva;* Tam. *Vilva.*

A small or medium-sized tree, commonly grown in Ceylon and other tropical countries for the fruit.

All parts of the plant are used either singly or with other drugs in several diseases. The juice of fresh leaves with honey is regarded as a febrifuge and laxative ; this, however, is seldom used now. The decoction of the leaves and root with pepper is a good cough mixture useful in chronic bronchitis, asthma and consumption. A strong decoction of the leaves is a common fomentation to rheumatic and painful swellings and neuralgia, and is also a good application for scabies and other skin complaints. The fresh flowers are bound over the eyes in ophthalmia.

Both the ripe and the unripe fruits are used in medicine. The unripe or half-ripe fruit is regarded as an astringent, digestive and stomachic and is used in dysentery and diarrhoea with debility of the mucous membrane ; it is particularly useful in chronic diarrhoea and dysentery of children. The ripe fruit is edible and is useful in diarrhoea, dysentery and dyspepsia. A syrup made by making 2 ounces of pulp with three or four ounces of water is laxative and is also useful in dyspepsia. In some parts of India, the half-ripe fruit and some curd with roasted rice is given for haemorrhoids.

The root bark in decoction is regarded as a corrective for deranged " air " (wata), and is also given in cases of melancholia, heart disease and fever.

Atalantia Missionis, Oliv., Eng. *The wild lime;* Sinh. *Pamburu;* Tam. *Kuruntu.*

A small tree, rather common, chiefly in the dry region of Ceylon. Its flowers are white and fragrant. It is also found in South India.

Atalantia zeylanica, Sinh. *Yakinaran;* Tam. *Peykuruntu.*

A much-branched bush, usually armed with very sharp, stout pines. A smaller variety is *A.rotundifolia.* They are rather common in the low-country of Ceylon. They have white sweet-scented flowers.

The leaf juice of these plants, especially of *A.zeylanica,* is used for the administration of pills. They are also regarded as useful in preventing ague.

Atalantia monophylla, Corr., No Sinhalese name; Sans. *Atavi-jambira;* Tam. *Perunkuruntu.*

A small tree or shrub, common in the dry region of Ceylon and in East Bengal and South India. Its wood is very hard, heavy, close-grained and yellow.

The decoction of the leaves is applied in itch and other skin complaints. The berries in the form of pickle are useful in whetting the appetite of patients convalescing from fever. The oil from the berries is a valuable application in chronic rheumatism and paralysis. The root is anti-spasmodic and stimulant. The juice of the fruit is anti-bilious.

The oil is prepared for use as a medicine by powdering the seeds, which are very aromatic when fresh, sprinkling them with sweet-oil and expressing ; the result is a dark-green, pleasant smelling oil, which communicates an agreeable warmth to the skin when rubbed on it. The seeds pressed by themselves yield no fatty oil, but the press-cloths are moistened with essential oil.

Feronia elephantum, Corr., Eng. *Wood apple;* Sinh. *Divul;* Sans. *Kapitha; Kapi-priya* (dear to monkeys); Tam. *Nila-vilam.*

A small spiny tree, 30-40 feet high and is a native of India and Ceylon. The globular or ovoid fruit is of the size of a large cricket ball, similar to the *Bael* fruit, but distinguished from it by the rough, woody, hard white shell. It is also called Elephant Apple, because the fruit which is edible is like an elephant's skin.

In medicinal properties it is similar to *Aegle marmelos.* The half-ripe fruit is very astringent and is prescribed with honey in dysentery. The pulp of the ripe fruit is edible and is useful in salivation, sore-throat and other affections of the gum and throat. A sherbet made out of it forms a cooling drink. The pulp is also applied externally in snake bite.

The transparent gummy substance which exudes from the stem when cut is used in bowel complaints and to relieve tenasmus ; powdered and mixed with honey it is given in dysentery and diarrhoea. When repeatedly treated with fuming nitric acid the gum gives mucic acid in abundant yield. It is believed that the gum answers better for mixing colours than gum-arabic. (Spons Encyc.)

The leaves are carminative and aromatic. The fruit is anti-scorbutic, astringent (when unripe) and refrigerant. The gum is demulcent.

Paramignya monophylla, Wight., Sinh. *Wellangiriya;* Tam. *Katillinsecham.*

A climbing shrub, rather common in the low country of Ceylon, principally in the dry regions, also in Burma and India. From the resemblance of its fruits to those of *Capparis zeylanica,* the Marathas call it *Karuwageti* (bitter Wageti). The root, which is the part used, has a scabrous brown bark and a bitter saline taste. It abounds in large crystals of calcium oxalate. It is used as a diuretic and alterative and is also given to cattle suffering from bloody urine or blood fluxes from the abdomen.

Ruta graveolens, Linn., Eng, *Herb of Grace, The Garden rue*, Sinh. *Arooda;* Sans. *Sadapa, Somalata;* Tam. *Arvada, Tirumuti-patchi.*

A small under-shrub with small glaucous leaves, commonly grown in gardens of Europe. It was introduced from the West into the East in the Middle Ages with all the superstitions attached to it. During the Middle Ages it was used like an amulet as protection against poison and as a preventive of epilepsy and vertigo. In Ceylon, it grows best in the hill country and in shaded spots at low and medium elevations.

In the East, the leaves are burnt and children suffering from catarrh are fumigated. Heating a few leaves crushed in a teaspoonful of oil and rubbing over the chest and forehead is a domestic remedy for infantile catarrh.

Oil of Rue is said to be distilled in France from *Ruta graveolens* with a yield of about 0.06%. In Algeria, however, two distinct oils of rue are distilled: "summer oil" from *Ruta montana* and "winter" oil from *Ruta bracteosa.* From *R. graveolens*, Haensel obtained 0.135% of an oil which was not identical with the ordinary oil of rue. Schimmel & Co. obtained 0.7% of oil from the dry herb of Smyrna. It congealed between $-7°$ and $-8°$, and was rich in methyl-heptyl ketone.

The two characteristic constituents of oil of rue are 2 ketones: methyl-*n*-heptyl ketone and methyl-*n*-nonyl ketone. The following have also been identified:—l-α-pinene, cineol, l-limonene and methyl salicylate. The blue fluorescence of the oil, which is occasionally observed, is traced to the presence of the methyl ester of methyl anthranilic acid. The following constants are from Gildemeister and Hoffmann, Volatile Oils II, 637 :—

	French oil	Algerian oil R. montana	Algerian oil R. brachteosa	Spanish oil
$D_{15°}$	0.8328-0.8437	0.8370-0.8381	0.8373-0.8446	0.834-0.847
α_D	$-0°40'$ to $+2°10'$	$+0°56'$	$+1°14'$ to $-5°$	$-1°$ to $+0°30'$
$N_D^{20°}$	1.430-1.434	1.4306-1.4322	1.430	1.4330
congealing pt.	5.8-10.8°			$-1.9°$

Characteristics for pure oil of rue are its low specific gravity and its solubility in 70% alcohol.

See also Power and Less, (J. Chem. Soc., 1902, *81*, 1585) Houben, (Ber., 1902, *35*, 3587). Haensel, (Abst. 1907, I, 65) obtained formic and butyric acids by saponification of German Oil of Rue.

Peganum Harmala, Linn., Syrian Rue, Sinh. *Rata-arooda* Sans. *Harmal;* Tam. *Shimai-azha-vanai-virai,*—is a glabrous bush.

Trimen does not mention either *Ruta graveolens* or or *P.Harmala.*

The seeds are regarded as narcotic, anodyne, emetic and emmenagogue, and act in large doses like ergot for which it is used as a substitute. It is also described as an alterative and purifying medicine in atrabilis, and also in diseases supposed to arise from cold humours such as palsy, lumbago, etc.; it is also said to stimulate the sexual system both in the male and the female, increasing the flow of milk and menses in the latter. For administration, a concentrated decoction is mixed with sweet oil and honey, or the crushed seeds are boiled in wine down to one-fourth of the original bulk of the latter, and the mixture strained. Gopal finds that the infusion or tincture acts as a stimulant emmenagogue and produces slight intoxication like *Cannabis indica.*

The seeds contain three alkaloids, harmaline, $C_{13}H_{14}ON_2$, isolated by Goebel (Ann. 1841, *38*, 363., harmine, $C_{13}H_{12}ON_2$, isolated by Fritsche (Ann),

1847, *64*, 365) and harmalol first prepared by O. Fischer (Ber., 1885 *18*, 400; 1889, *22*, 637; 1897, *30*, 2481).

Harmaline crystallises from alcohol or benzene in colourless prisms, melting with decomposition at 250°. Harmine crystallises from methyl alcohol in colourless rhombic prisms m.p. 259°.

The constitution of these alkaloids has been worked out by O. Fischer and his colleagues and more recently by Perkin and Robinson. (See Ber., 1885, *18*, 403; 1897, *30*, 2482; 1912, *45*, 1934; 1914, *47*, 99 and J. Chem. Soc., 1912, *101*, 1778; 1919, *115*, 967; 1921, *119*, 1604, 1617; 1922, *121*, 1872.)

P. Harmala has been used as a remedy for tape-worm in man. Flury states (Arch. exp. path. Pharm., 1910, *64*, 105) that harmaline has an anthelmintic action, probably by paralysing the musculature of the parasites and that harmine, harmaline and tetrahydroharmine have a paralysing action on frogs, whilst apoharmine causes increased reflex irritability and tetanus. In warm-blooded animals harmine and harmaline cause convulsions, increase of saliva, interference of respiration and depression of temperature.

Gunn and Marshall (Proc. Roy. Soc. Edin., 1920, *40*, 140) have found that harmine and harmaline are useful in malaria. (For a short account, see Henry's Plant Alkaloids.)

Murraya Koenigii, Spr., Sinh. *Karapincha;* Sans. *Saurabinimba* (fragrant Neem); Tam. *Karuveppilai.*

It is a small tree with a dark-grey bark. It grows in the moist regions of India. It is familiar as the curry-leaf plant.

The leaves, bark and root are tonic and stomachic. The root is also slightly purgative. The herb is a good remedy for dysentery at the outset. Roasted leaves are given for vomiting. The leaves are much used as an ingredient in sauces and are given in decoction with bitters as a febrifuge.

The fruits yield upon distillation 0.76% of an oil (Ber. von Roure-Bertrand Fils, April 1903, 35 and Gild. & Hoffmann, II, 648) with a neroli-like odour and a pepper-like taste, but leaves an agreeable sense of coolness on the tongue. It has the following constants :—$D_{13°}$ 0.872, $\alpha_D -27°24'$, n_D 1.487, b.p. 173-174°.

By treatment with ether and drying, a greenish black resin was obtained in 7.5% yield. This resin extracted with water and evaporated gave a small residue equivalent to 3% of the resin. The aqueous extract was slightly acid and reduced Fehling's solution. On acidifying with sulphuric acid a similarly prepared alcoholic extract, a few granular crystals were obtained, which were supposed to be a glucoside and named Koenigin (Pharm. Ind.)

Murraya exotica, Linn., Sinh. *Etteriya;* Sans. *Ekangi.*

A small graceful tree with a smooth yellowish-white, fibrous bark, and white, scented flowers. The variety *M.buxifolia* is a more floriferous shrub, much grown in gardens for its beauty and sweet scent. They are found throughout India, and in China, Australia and the Pacific Islands.

It is a tonic stomachic like *M.Koenigii.*. It is said to be aromatic, refrigerant, digestive and beneficial in rheumatic fever, cough, giddiness, hysteria, thirst and burning of the feet.

In Burma, the fragrant bark is more universally used as a cosmetic than sandalwood.

De Vrij separated from the flowers a glucoside named Murrayin, $C_{18}H_{22}O_{10}$.

The Genus Zanthoxylum, consists of about 80 species but only a very few are found in Ceylon. *Z.tetraspermum* is found in Ceylon, chiefly in the mountain zone 3000-6000 feet high, where it is rather common. It is stimulant, astringent and digestive and is prescribed in dyspepsia and some forms of diarrhoea.

Z.Hamiltonianum and *Z.Budrunga* are the "*Katukeena*" of the Sinhalese (Sans. *Tumburu;* Tam. *Rhetsamaram*). Their fruits resemble coriander from which they are with difficulty distinguished. Its properties are similar to those of *Z. tetraspermum*.

Giacosa and Monari (Gazetta, *17*, 362; Abst., 1888, 167) obtained an oil by extracting the bark of *Z.senagalese* (artar root). From this oil a solid separated which contained no nitrogen and when purified had a white micaceous appearance (m.p. 120-125°), and gave a purple colouration with chloroform and sulphuric acid. Sufficient material was not in hand for a complete investigation. The bark after treatment with petroleum gave on prolonged boiling with alcohol a brownish extract, from which on addition of alkali, a yellowish solid was obtained. This consists of two alkaloids, one of which is amorphous and insoluble in water and the other crystalline and soluble. The former was not further examined. The latter gave the following crystalline derivatives: hydrochloride, nitrate, and platinichloride. The in-soluble alkaloid produces muscular irritation and coagulation of myrosin and physiological disturbances analogous to those of veratrine. The compounds were not analysed. Giacosa and Soave (Gaz., *19*, 303; Abst., 1890,918) find that the crystalline alkaloid is not a constant constituent of the bark. The amorphous one was obtained by extraction of the root with 94% alcohol, concentrating the solution to a syrup, adding alkali, extracting with ether to which HCl is added after concentration, when the hydrochloride crystallises out. This alkaloid is named artarine and is found to the extent of 0.4%. Other salts and some colour reactions are described in the paper.

Z.ochroxylum from Central and South America contain, according to Leprince (Abst., 1912, ii, 479) two alkaloids, α and β -xantherines, belonging to the group of berberine: two crystalline neutral substances α - and β -xanthoxylins, and a mixture of ethereal and fatty oils.

α -antherine, $C_{24}H_{23}O_6N$, m.p. 186° from benzene, goes yellow on exposure to air. The hydrochloride of β -xantherine differs from that of the compound in that it is very soluble in water. The "fatty" substances distil in vacuo without decomposition and are for the most part unsaponified on treatment with alcoholic potash. They have a sharp burning anaesthetic taste and act as analgesiac. α -xantherine has a paralytic action on the intercardial nervous system.

Jowett and Pyman (J. Chem. Soc., 1913, *103*, 290) have investigated the alkaloids of *Z.brachyacanthum* from Queensland. The chief alkaloid of the bark is a quaternary base whose chloride is identical with l-canadine methochloride. This is the first record of the isolation from a plant of a substance containing an asymmetric nitrogen atom.

The occurrence of crystalline, neutral principles of indifferent members of the genus *Zanthoxylum* has been established and these substances have been shown to be lactones (Bocquillon, Abst., 1917, i, 276)

Ligroin extracts from *Z.carolianum* carixanthide, $C_{12}H_{24}O$, m.p. 285°, while *Z.carolianum* gives carolixanthide, m.p. 119°. The occurrence in the seeds of *Z.piperitum* of the crystalline substance (m.p.80°) isolated by Stenhouse (Ann., 1854, *89*, 251; 1857, *104*, 236) is confirmed as well as the presence of α - and β -xanthoxylin, m.p., 162° and 187° respectively in the seeds of *Z. ochroxylum* as recorded by Leprince. All these substances are accompanied by fixed or volatile oils.

Dieterle (Arch. Pharm., 1919, *257*, 260; Abst., 1920, i, 42) has obtained in about 0.25% yield a crystalline substance, Xanthosterol, $C_{23}H_{40}O$, by extracting the bark of *Z.Budrunga* with ligroin. It melts at 213-214°. It is an alcohol related to lupeol and alstol. Some colour reactions are described. He also mentions the presence of an alkaloid which he proposes to study later.

Schimmel & Co. (Chem. Zentr., 1907, i, 1413; Abst. 1907, i, 782) have obtained a yellowish green ethereal oil from *Z. aubertia* from Reunion. It has a distinct odour of parsley but does not contain phellandrene. It gave the following values :—D_{15} 0.9052, $\alpha_D -62°10'$, acid number 1.3, ester number 7.3.

The composition of the essential oils of *Z.aubertia* and *Z.alatum* has been investigated by Semmler and Schossberger (Ber., 1911, *44*, 2885; Abst., 1911, i, 1002). The oil of the former was divided into three fractions: (1) b.p., 70-80° at 16 mm. pressure, comprised 2-3% and had D_{20} 0.8248, n_D 1.4977, $\alpha_D + 30°$; probably an aliphatic terpene. (2) b.p., 115-130° (same pressure) comprised 80-90%. The purified material gave the following constants :—b.p., (9 mm.) 119-123°, $D_{20°}$ 0.8781, n_D 1.499, $\alpha_D -58°$. It contains a sesquiterpene evodene of the same type as limene and eugenol methyl ether which was 40-60% of the crude oil (3) solid, m.p., 85°, which is phloracetophenone dimethyl ether $C_{10}H_{12}O_4$.

The oil of *Z.alatum* gave the following fractions (1) b.p., 50-60° comprised 80% of the crude oil, is probably l-sabinene but is provisionally termed Xanthoxylene; constants D_{20} 0.84, n_D 1.4746, $\alpha_D -26°$. (2) 5-10% of the crude oil yields two semicarbazones, m.p., 210° and 221°; the former corresponds to cuminaldehyde (3) the third fraction consists of phloroacetophenene dimethyl ether.

Peckolt (Gildemeister & Hoffmann, 11, 631) obtained from the leaves an oil with a rue like odour and a specific gravity of 0.894.

According to Helbing (Gildemeister & Hofmann, 11, 627) the seeds of *Z.Hamiltonianum* yielded 3.8 to 5% of a colourless volatile oil with a specific gravity of 0.840. Its smell is reminiscent of a mixture of geranium and bergamot oils.

There are several species of Citrus used in medicine. *Citrus Aurantium (var. C. sinensis)* Sinh. *Panidodan;* Tam. *Narankai,* —is a small tree or shrub, supposed to be indigenous to North India.

C.acida (C.aurantifolia), lime, Sinh. *Debi;* Tam. *Dhasikai,*—is a small spiny tree, cultivated in all tropical countries for its acid, juicy fruit. It is used for flavouring and culinary purposes and is applied externally for snake-bites.

C.limonum, Sinh. *Naran;* Tam. *Kidanar-atankai.*

There are several varieties of *naran ; Heen-naran, Jama-naran;* the juice of the former is very frequently used in medicine, for " purifying minerals ", grinding some stock pills, with honey and rock-salt for rheumatism, sciatica, etc.

C.decumana, Eng. *Shaddock, Pomelo,* Sinh. *Jambola;* Tam. *Jamblica.*

A small tree 25-30 feet high, native of tropical Asia and cultivated for its fruit. It is not used in medicine.

For information regarding the Essential Oils from this family, see Gildemeister & Hoffmann and other works on essential oils.

SIMARUBACEAE

Ailanthus malabarica, D.C., Sinh. *Kumbalu, or Walbiling;* Sans. *Mahanimba.*

A large tree, common in many parts of India and in the moist low country forests of Ceylon. *A.excelsa* of which *A.malabarica* is a variety[l] is not mentioned by Trimen.

The bark and leaves are used in India for debility after childbirth. An infusion of the bark and leaves is also given in bronchitis and asthma. On incision, the bark yields a dark-coloured soft resin known in India as *Matti-phal*, which in time hardens into a brittle resin with a strong balsamic odour. It is used in dysentery.

The leaves of *A.glandulosa* (not found in Ceylon) have been examined by Perkin and Wood (J. Chem. Soc. 1898,*73*, 381). The leaves obtained from Cyprus were finely ground and extracted with boiling water. The colouring matters were found to be principally quercetin and ellagic acid. Gallic and gallotannic acids were also found.

Balanites Roxburghii, Planch., Sinh. and Sans. *Ingudi;* Tam. *Nanjundi,*—is a shrub met with in the dry parts of India. It is not found in Ceylon. The dried fruits are imported from India. An oil prepared from the seeds is used by the Hindus in the initiation ceremony of the young student. It is used in medicine as an application for ocline. The bark, unripe fruits and leaves are pungent, bitter, purgative and anthelmintic and are used in worms in children.

Samadera indica, Gaertn., Eng. *Neepa-bark tree;* Sinh. *Samadara;* Tam. *Neepa;* Sans. *Lokhandi.*

It is a tree 30 to 35 feet high, indigenous to the Western Indian Peninsula and also rather common in the forests of the moist low country of Ceylon.

The bark and seeds are very bitter and the former is used as a febrifuge. The drug may be used as a substitute for quassia. The bruised leaves are externally applied in erysipelas and the seeds are worn round the neck as a preventive of asthma and chest affections. An oil extracted from the kernels is a good application in rheumatism.

In 1872 De Vrij expressed from the seeds 33% of a light yellow bitter oil, which contains according to Oudemans, 84% of olein and 16% of palmitin and stearin. The bitter principle, samaderin, or quassin, was yellowish, amorphous and soluble in water and alcohol. It had been obtained by Tonningen in 1858 from the seed and bark in white scales which became yellow with nitric or hydrochloric acid and violet-red with sulphuric acid. (see Year-book of Pharm., 1886, 196).

More recently the plant has been chemically and pharmacologically investigated by van der Marck (Ned. Tijd. Pharm., *12*, 296; Abst., 1901, ii, 71 and Arch. Pharm., 1909, *239*, 96; Abst., 1901, ii, 334). In the papers the author gives a morphological description of the drug and an account of the chemical investigation. Most of the substances isolated were obtained in very small yield :— (1) The seeds give 63% of a fatty oil, containing 88% triolein, 8% tripalmitin and 4% tristearin. (2) a proteid soluble in alcohol and in water and containing 18% nitrogen. (3) sucrose (4) a reducing sugar (5) inositol (6) a crystalline bitter substance. From the bark (1) the same bitter principle (2) a crystalline bitter substance, probably an anthraquinone derivative (3) a phloroglucotannin (4) ellagotannic acid (5) a tannic acid closely resembling tannin. From the wood, 2 bitter substances, one closely allied to quassin. The bitter substance occurring in both the seeds and the bark melts at 255°, $[\alpha]_D$ + 250°, and formula $C_{29}H_{34}D_{11}$.

CUCURBITACEAE

Citrullus Colocynthus, Schrad., Sinh. *Yak-komadu;* Sans. *Indravaruna, Vishala;* Tam. *Paykkomaddi.*

It grows in India, Arabia, Western Asia, North and Tropical Africa and the Mediterranean countries. "The plant is not cultivated in Ceylon and the fruit used is that of the wild plant and differs much in size from the colocynth obtained from the Mediterranean for pharmaceutical purposes." (Trimen).

It is described by Sanskrit writers as bitter, acrid and cathartic. In moderate doses colocynth is a drastic hydrogogue, cathartic and diuretic; in large doses an emetic and gastro-intestinal irritant. In small doses it also acts as an expectorant and alterative. It is useful in biliousness, constipation, fever, worms and other cases requiring purgatives. The juice of the fruit mixed with sugar is a household remedy in dropsy. The seed oil is used for blackening grey hairs. Colocynth is rarely employed alone but is generally given with other purgatives and carminatives.

The oil of colocynth seeds obtained by extraction with carbon tetrachloride has been investigated by Grimaldi and Prussia (Abst. 1909, ii, 426) D_{15} 0.9289, Sap. Val. 191.7, Iod. Val. (Hubl) 120.37., It has slight drying properties and is similar to those obtained from other *Cucurbitaceae*.

Colocynthin and other substances from the dried pealed fruit have been investigated by various workers. Power and Moore (J. Chem. Soc. 1910, 97, 99) have examined the constituents of Turkish colocynth. (This paper contains a resume of earlier work on the subject.) The ground pulp was completely extracted with hot alcohol and the extract on steam distillation gave a small quantity of oil (not investigated). From the portion non-volatile in steam the following substances were isolated: (1) Citrullol, $C_{22}H_{36}O_2(OH)_2$, crystallising from hot pyridine, m.p., 285-290°, an amorphous substance which is a very weak base, from which no crystalline derivative was prepared. It possesses an extremely bitter taste and represents one of the purgative principles of the fruit.

(2) α -elaterin, m.p., 232°, $[\alpha]_D$-68.9°, a small amount of, hentriacontane $C_{31}H_{64}$, m.p. 68°, a phytosterol, $C_{27}H_{46}O$ m.p., 160-162°, glucose and a mixture of fatty acids.

The seeds were also examined by them from which they obtained an enzyme which hydrolyses β -glucosides, and an oil. The authors also conclude that the so-called colocynthin and colocynthitin as well as the other products obtained from colocynth by previous investigators consisted of mixtures of a very indefinite character and that the amount of glucosidic substances contained in the fruit is extremely small, and further that the purgative action of the drug is due at least to two principles, one alkaloidal and the other some non-basic principle or principles contained in the resin obtained from the pulp.

Citrullus vulgaris, Schrad., or Cucurbita Citrullus, linn., Eng. *Water melon;* Sinh. *Komadu;* Sans. *Chayapula, Kuttoowombi.*

A plant indigenous to Tropical Africa but is cultivated throughout the East. The distinction between the water melon and the cultivated form of *C.Colocynthus* is very small.

The juice is useful in quenching thirst and is also used as an antiseptic in typhus fever. With cumin and sugar the juice is used as a cooling drink in strangury and affections of the urinary organs, such as gonorrhoea etc., and also in hepatic congestion and intestinal catarrh. The seeds of the water melon are of interest as being one of the four cold cucurbitaceous seeds of the Ancients. In India these are *Cucumis utilissimus, Citrullus vulgaris, Benincasa cerifera* and *Cucumis melo.*

Power and Salway (J. Am. Chem. Soc., 1910, 32, 360) have examined the oil obtained from the seeds of the water melon grown in the U.S.A. The oil was extracted by hydraulic pressure of the kernels freed from the shells. The entire seed ground and extracted with ligroin gave 19% of fatty oil. The oil extracted in this way was also examined. The expressed oil was yellow and devoid of fluorescence.

	Expressed Oil	Extracted Oil
Sp. Gr. 20°/20°	0.9233	0.9219
Acid Value	3.9	3.6
Saponification Val.	191.8	189.9
Iodine Value	121.1	121.8

The oil gave a substance, m.p., 163-164° (probably a phytosterol) linoleic, oleic, palmitic and stearic acids. The " press-cake " contained oil, a phytosterol, a new alcohol, cucurbitol $C_{24}H_{40}O_4$ melting at 260° with decomposition. This alcohol is not present in the shells.

The resin both from the kernel and the shell of the seed is inocuous.

Lagenaria vulgaris, Seringe. Eng. *Bottle Gourd;* Sinh. *Diya-labu;* Sans. *Alabu;* Tam. *Sorakai.*

A creeper found wild and cultivated all over India. It is cultivated for its fruit which is a popular cheap vegetable.

The seed and the pulp of the fruit are used in medicine. The pulp is used as a cathartic. The seeds yield an oil used as an application for the head to relieve headache. Externally the pulp is used as a cooling application on the shaved head in delirium and to the soles in " burning of the feet." The leaves are purgative and are recommended to be taken in the form of decoction for jaundice.

The poisonous properties of the bitter variety have been noticed and the symptoms observed are similar to those after poisoning by elaterium or colocynth.

Cucumis pubescens. Sinh. *Gon-kekiri* and *Cucumis trigonus, Roxb., Pseudocolocynth;* Tam. *Metukku;* Sans. *Vishala.*

These are common and grow on waste ground in the low-country of Ceylon. The fruit which is bitter is not eaten but is used sometimes in the same way as *Citrullus vulgaris.* The seeds are said to be cooling and are applied in the form of a paste with the juice of *Cynodon dactylon* to herpetic swellings. The root in decoction is used as a purgative and is said to be milder in effect than the pulp of the fruit and causes less irritation.

Naylor and Chappel (Pharm. Journ. 1907, 79, 117; Abst. 1907, ii, 807) have obtained from *C.trigonus* a principle identical with or closely related to colocynthin. (see under *Citrullus colocynthus*)

Cucurbita Pepo or Benincasa cerifera, Savi., Eng. *Ash pumpkin.* Sinh. *Puhul or Alu-puhul;* Sans. *Kushmanda.*

This plant is cultivated for its fruit which is used as a vegetable; the pulp is also candied. It has important medicinal uses, the seeds, the fruit and the fruit juice being the parts used.

The fruit is nutritive, tonic and diuretic. In phthisis, pearl-ash is administered with the fresh juice. It is used as an antidote for many vegetable poisons and in mercurial and alcoholic poisoning. It is said to be a highly nutritious food in wasting diseases such as consumption. It is an ingredient in certain preparations for phthisis, asthma, heart disease, etc. It is also said to be used with success in diabetes, four ounces of the juice with 100 grains each of saffron and the bran of red rice are given morning and evening, and a strict diet enjoined.

Power and Salway (Journ. Am. Chem. Soc., 1910, 32, 346) have made a chemical examination of the seeds "which have been recognized for several decades by the United States Pharmacoepia under the title of Pepo, and are regarded as an efficient and harmless taenifuge." The seeds do not contain an alkaloid. On extraction with ligroin the entire seeds gave 34.3% of fatty oil. Oil was also prepared by expressing the kernels freed from shell with a 19.3% yield.

	Expressed Oil	Oil extracted by ligroin.
Sp. Gr. 20°/20°	0.9220	0.9212
Acid Value	3.4	3.5
Sap. Value	189.4	189.0
Iodine Val.	119.7	119.6

On saponification the oil gave the following acids :— Palmitic, stearic, oleic and linoleic. The press cake gave a quantity of fatty oil, soluble protein products, sugar, a very small quantity of salicylic acid, a resinous material and a new monocarboxylic acid $C_{25}H_{51}O$. COOH, m.p.99° The shells on extraction with hot alcohol gave a fatty oil. similar to the expressed oil, sugar and a small quantity of resinous matter.

The authors also examined the physiological properties. The pure expressed oil of the seeds was administered in doses of 30cc., under the usual conditions of a restricted diet, to two dogs suffering from tapeworm. Castor oil was given after an interval of several hours but in neither case was any tapeworm found in the excreta. Negative results were also obtained with the resin. Experiments on children too proved negative. Power and Solway are of opinion that " the remedial value of pumpkin seeds cannot be considered such as to justify their recognition by a national pharmacoepia."

For " Contents of Cribiferous Vessels of Cucurbita Pepo " see Zacharias, Abst., 1884, 1067.

Cucurbita maxima. Eng. *Red Gourd;* Sinh. *Wattakka, Ratalabu;* Sans. *Punya-latha, Dadhipala.*

This is a climbing or creeping gourd, bearing large, round, smooth fruits which are generally flattened at both ends. Emptied of the pulp and seeds, the shell becomes very hard, light and durable and is commonly used in the Tropics for baskets, etc. It is cultivated in all parts of India and Ceylon and is frequently found on the roofs of houses. The fruit is a popular vegetable.

The juice of the fruit is given with milk and honey at the commencement of bilious fevers. The seeds are given with sugar in tapeworm—given at bedtime followed by castor oil in the morning. They are also used as a diuretic in gonorrhoea. The pulp is used as a poultice for boils, carbuncles, etc. and in pneumonia.

Osborne and Campbell (Journ. Am. Chem. Soc., 1896, 18, 609) have found the protein edestin in the pulp. The composition of the seed oil has been examined by Baughman and Jamieson (Journ. Amer. Chem.Soc., 1920, 42, 152). The expressed oil had Sp. gr. 25°/25° 0.9179, Ref. Index (25°) 1.4714, Iod. val. 121.0, Sap. val., 191.5, etc. and the glycerides of the following acids were present:— Palmitic 13%, stearic 6%, arachidic 0.04%, oleic 37%, and linolic 44% and 1% of unsaponifiable matter.

Trichosanthes dioica. Roxb. Eng. *Snake gourd or Club gourd;* Sinh. *Pathola;* Sans. *Chichinda;* Tam. *Podivilangu or Podalangai.*

A quick growing annual gourd, native of China and Malaya, bearing long green or greenish white fruits. In the immature state the fruit is used as a vegetable, particularly popular for convalescing patients.

Trichosanthes cucumerina, Linn. Sinh. *Dummella;* Sans. *Patola;* Tam. *Katup-pepudal.*

This is largely used in medicine, especially in fever, and is almost a constant ingredient in decoctions for fevers. The root is purgative, tonic and anthelmintic. The juice of the leaves is emetic and that of the root purgative. The stalk in decoction is expectorant. According to the authors of Pharm. Ind., the febrifuge action appears to depend on its purgative properties.

Trichosanthes palmata, Roxb. Sinh. *Titta-hondala;* Sans. *Mahakala;* Tam. *Koratti, Shavari-paspam.*

The fruit is a violent hydrogogue cathartic. The fruit powdered and mixed with oil is used for offensive discharges from the ear. The dried shell is powdered and smoked in a pipe, like tabacco, for asthma. The oil of the seed is dropped into the ear for otorrhoea; it has also been found useful in hemicrania. The root is poisonous and is used in the pneumonia of cattle.

The rind and pulp of the fruit contain an amorphous bitter principle which gives an abundant precipitate with tannin and reduces Fehling's Solution. (Pharm. Ind. Tschirch Abst., 1893, i, 42) extracted the succulent part of the fruit, *Trichosanthes pubera* (not found in Ceylon) with ether (obtaining a red pigment) and then the residue with alcohol which gave a green pigment, tricosanthin. It was purified by dissolving in hydrochloric acid and precipitating with water. It is a black powder and its solution in hydrochloric acid is blue.

Momordica charantia, Linn. Sinh. *Karawila;* Sans. *Ugralata or Kandira;* Tam. *Pavakai, Nutipak.*

A rather slender vine, bearing an ovoid, warty gourd, bright orange-yellow when ripe, and commonly cultivated in the Tropics as a vegetable.

The leaves are used externally for skin affections of parasitic origin. A poultice made of the leaves and those of *Cassia alata* is used in Malaya in skin diseases of children. The juice of the fresh leaves is given to children as a mild purgative but is not unattended with danger; the antidote is ghee and rice. Night blindness is said to be cured by the application, round the orbit, of the leaf juice in which black pepper is ground. The root is febrifuge and the seed anthelmintic. The fruit is considered tonic, stomachic and cooling and is used in rheumatism, gout and diseases of the spleen and liver. It is supposed to purify the blood. When ripe it is a drastic purgative.

A bitter glucoside soluble in water but insoluble in ether, a yellow acid and a resin have been found to occur in the plant.

Momordica cochinchienensis, Spr., vel Diocia. Sinh. *Tumba-karawila;* Sans. *Karkataka Vahasa;* Tam. *Tumpai or Paluppakai.*

A small oblong green, warty-looking gourd commonly used as a vegetable (usually for convalescents). The tender shoots and leaves are also edible. The wild variety is bitter but under cultivation it loses much of its bitterness.

It is a domestic remedy for sores caused by the urine of the house lizard. When mixed with pepper, coconut milk and sandalwood and applied externally it is a useful remedy for cephalalgia. The powder of the root applied to the skin renders it soft and lessens perspiration.

According to the Pharmacopoeia Indica, the seed kernels give 43.7% of a slightly greenish oil when treated with petroleum ether. The oil possessed very powerful siccative properties. The fatty acids from it melted at 48-49.° A slightly bitter glucoside was also obtained.

Luffa acutangula, Roxb. Sinh. *Vatakolu or Dara-vatakolu;* Sans. *Koshataki;* Tam. *Pekan-kai.*

A gourd with several sharp, longitudinal ridges, it is commonly used in the tender state as a vegetable. The plant is an annual and is commonly grown in India, Ceylon, etc.

The fruit is demulcent, diuretic and nutritive. An infusion of the ripe fruit is administered as an emetic and purgative. The seeds, particularly the ripe ones are emetic and purgative. The oil from them is used in cutaneous complaints ; its chemical nature is, however, not known. The root is laxative. The drug is recommended in enlargements of the spleen. The juice of the leaves is used as an external application to sores and the bites of venomous animals. The pulp of the fruit is administered internally in cases of bites of animals to cause vomiting and purging just as colocynth. The dried fruit is powdered and made into a snuff for those suffering from jaundice.

Luffa aegyptica, Eng. *Loofa or Spone gourd;* Sinh. *Niyan-vatakolu;* Sans. *Raja-koshataki;* Tam. *Pikku, Pichukku:*

This is an annual gourd. By wetting the fruit in water, a fibrous inter-lacing network is obtained, which is commonly used as a bath-sponge, manufactured largely in Japan for export. The seeds which give a reddish-brown oil are said to be emetic and cathartic. It is generally similar to *L.acutangula.* It is one of the plants used in India for the preparation of pearl-ash.

Luffa echinata. Roxb., Sinh. *Dedali;* Sans. *Devadali, etc.* It has to be used with caution. A case of poisoning with symptoms resembling those of cholera after the administration of one fruit as a purgative is mentioned in Pharm. Indica.

Cephalandra indica, Naud. Sinh. *Kowakka;* Sans. *Vimbaja, Tundika, Vimboshaa;* Tam. *Kovvai.*

It is a perennial herb of which the leaves, root, fruit and bark are used. The fresh juice of the leaves is applied to bites of animals. The leaves are bruised and applied to the wounds caused by snake-bites (Roberts). Attygalle, however, states that the fresh root is used for this purpose. Mixed with ghee, the leaf is applied to sores and skin diseases. The green fruit is chewed to cure sores on the tongue. It is also used as an adjunct to metallic preparations for diabetes.

A chemical examination of the tubers is given in the Pharm. Indica. The authors have detected alkaloids, a resin insoluble in acids, a resin insoluble in alkaline carbonates but easily soluble in sodium hydroxide but less readily in ammonia and starch; no tannin matter was found.

Zanonia indica, Linn. Sinh. *Wal-rasakinda;* Sans. *Dhirga-patra, Kuntali,* Eng. *Bandolier fruit,*—is met with in Assam, Bengal, Ceylon and the Malabar coast.

In Ceylon it is used as a febrifuge. It is described as "cold", aperient and beneficial in asthma and cough. The leaf beaten with milk and butter is used as an application to allay the nervous irritation of boils. The fresh juice is said to be an efficacious antidote to venomous bites.

Zehneria umbellata, Thwaites. Sinh. *Kavudu-kekiri;* Sans. *Karivivalli, Gumthi;* Tam. *Peyppudal*—is extremely variable in the shape of its leaves. They are used externally in skin diseases. The root is stimulating and invigorating. It does not appear to have had a place in the Sanskrit Materia Medica.

Corallocarpus epigaeus, Hook.f. Sinh. *Gopalanga;* Sans. *Patala-garada; Mahamoola;* Tam. *Kollan-kovaik-kizhangu.*

A climber having a very large turnip shaped root, hence the Sanskrit name.

It is regarded as a valuable remedy for rheumatism. It is used in the later stages of dysentery and old venereal complaints, and usually administered in the form of a powder, which is of a very pale colour. It has been suggested by the authors of the Pharm. Ind. that this drug should be more carefully examined.

Dymock and others examined an aqueous extract after removing mucilage by treatment with alcohol. Extraction with chloroform or amyl alcohol gave a white amorphous mass soluble in water and spirit but very slightly soluble in ether. This is the bitter principle which is identical with bryonin, the bitter principle of the bryony root. On hydrolysis with dilute sulphuric acid it gives glucose and two amorphous bodies, bryoretin soluble in ether, and hydrobryotin, insoluble in ether but soluble in alcohol.

$$C_{48}H_{80}O_{19} + 2\,H_2O = \underset{\text{(Hydrobryotin)}}{C_{21}H_{37}O_8} + \underset{\text{(Bryoretin)}}{C_{21}H_{35}O_7} + C_6H_{12}O_6$$

Bryonia lacinosa, Linn. Sinh. *Kemvel;* Sans. *Baja.*

Its juice is given with milk, honey or sugar in bilious attacks and in the commencements of fevers when there is flatulence and constipation. It clears out the bowels and is often sufficient when the symptoms are due to overeating.

There are two plants in Europe which yield bryony ot, which was formerly, but is no longer used medicin- y. They are *Bryonia alba* and *Bryonia dioica,* both of iich are indigenous to the greater part of Europe. These o species are not found in Ceylon. The recorded works bryony root are:—Konnick and Marquart (Ber. 1870, 281) and (Ber. 1871, 4, 921); Sacc (Compt. rend. 94, 26, Abst. 1882, ii, 884), examined Uruguay bryony and und pectic acid, lignose, inulin and glucose.

Johannson (Abst. 1885, i, 606) showed that bryonin sembles colocynthin in its reactions. Etard (Compt. nd., *114*, 364; Ber., 1892, 25, 286) isolated bryonan, $_{20}H_{42}$, flat needles melting at 69°, boiling at 400°, om *B.dioica.* Masson (J. pharm. Chim. 1893, 27, 300 bst., 1893, i, 424) isolated bryonin, $C_{34}H_{48}O_9$ as a white, ery bitter amorphous powder, which gave on hydrolysis ith dilute sulphuric acid, glucose and a resinous subs- ince, bryogenin, $C_{28}H_{38}O_4$ m.p. 210°; A resin, ryoresin, was also isolated as a red amorphous ubstance, softening at 15° and becoming liquid at 50°.

Power and Moore have made much fuller investigation J.Chem. Soc., 1911, 99, 937) of the roots of *B.dioica.* They solated the following:—an enzyme in the form of a light orown powder which hydrolysed amygdalin and salicin; ı small quantity of a pale yellow essential oil; a small quantity of a colourless crystalline neutral substance, m.p. 220-222° of the probable formula $C_{20}H_{30}O_5$; an amorphous glucoside which on hydrolysis gave sugar and a brown resin; an amorphous alkaloidal principle, weakly basic and incapable of forming salts; a phytosterol, $C_{27}H_{46}O$, m.p. 137°; a new dihydric alcohol, bryonol, $C_{22}H_{34}O_2(OH)_2$, m. p. 210-212°; oleic, linolic, palmitic and stearic acids. They infer that " bryonin " of previous investigators is a complex mixture.

The crystalline neutral substance and the glucoside were found to be inactive physiologically. The 'alkaloid' produces slight purgation. The resinous material of the root also produces marked purgation.

Mukia scabrella, Arn. Sinh. *Heen-kekeri;* Sans. *Ahilekana;* Tam. *Mosumusikai,*—is found in the Tropics of the Old World generally.

The leaves are used as an expectorant and for this reason used as an ingredient in preparations for chronic diseases with cough as a predominant symptom. It is also a mild cathartic. The seeds in decoction are sudorific. The root similarly prepared is used in flatulence and when masticated relieves toothache.

Cucumis melo, Eng. *Musk melon.* Sinh. *Kekiri or Piti-kekiri;* Sans. *Kharvya;* Tam. *Velapalam or Molampalam.*

This is a plant used to a hot dry climate. The fruit' the interior of which is of a somewhat floury consistency (hence the second Sinhalese name), has a strong pleasant odour. It is the most important species of the genus, *Cucumis,* and is extensively cultivated for its fruit en the sandy banks of Indian rivers.

The flattened seeds yield 30% of a sweet, light, thin, tdible oil. In fact the seeds of most of the *Cucurbitaceae* contain oil but the only kinds which are utilized to any considerable extent are those of *Cucumis melo* and *Citrullus vulgaris.* The supply of melon oil in India and Ceylon is not extensive because the fruits are not allowed to ripen. The oil is also used in the soap industry.

Medicinally *C.melo* is regarded as cooling, diuretic and nutritive. It is used in painful micturition and suppression of urine, this property being found in the seed oil.

Forti (Ber. 1891, 24R, 76) isolated from the seeds a substance, melting at about 160° and having the same composition as ordinary cholesterin.

Cucumis sativus, Eng. *Cucumber.* Sinh. *Pipingna;* Sans. *Trapusha;* Tam. *Pipingkai,*—is cultivated in semi-dry districts. The fruit belongs to the same genus as the European cucumber and is used as a vegetable and a salad.

The seeds and root possess the same properties as most members of the *Cucumis* family. The seeds yield an oil similar to those from other members of the genus.

Cucumis utilissimus (not found in Ceylon) has been investigated by Green (Abst., 1884, ii, 63) who found trypsin in the fruit. The juice of the fruit dissolves boiled white of egg; the boiled juice does not act in this way. The action is not due to microbes since the addition of thymol does not prevent the action. Salt water dissolves more of the ferment than pure water. Like papain, the enzyme resembles trypsin rather than pepsin. The change proceeds as follows :—

Coagulated albumen—> peptone—> leucine.

BURSERACEAE

Balsamodendron Mukul, Hook. Sinh. *Gugul or Rata-dummala;* Sans. *Gugulu;* Tam. *Vellaipolam.*

There are several varieties of this used in Ayurvedic medicine. Their gums under the general name of frankincense are used for fumigating sick rooms. The plants are indigenous to Persia from where large quantities of the gum are exported.

Canarium zeylanicum, Sinh. *Kekuna;* Tam. *Pakkilipai.*

A very large much-branched tree, common in the moist low country of Ceylon. It flowers from May to September. The whole tree is fragrant when bruised. A beautifully clear, fragrant, balsamic gum-resin (much used for fumigation), like the *Elemi* of commerce, flows from the bark. The oily seeds are eaten. The oil is also used by the poor for lamps.

Canarium commune, Linn., Eng. *the Java almond;* Sinh. *Ratakekuna,*—is a native of Malaya and has been introduced to Ceylon before 1824. The fruit is much larger than that of *C.zeylanicum* and the seeds form a good substitute for almond.

The oleo-resins of many species of *Canarium* have been studied. *C.luzonicum* of the Phillipines is found to give the maximum flow of resin when the tree produces new leaves. One of these large trees yielded in two months 22 kgm. of the resin (*Elemi* of commerce). This yielded 20-36% of oil on steam distillation. For further particulars, see Gildemeister & Hoffmann, Voeatile Oils iii, 131 et seq. and Phil. Journal of Science. 1907, 2, 1.

MELIACEAE

Aglaia Roxburghiana, Miq. Sinh. *Puwangu;* Sans. *Priyangu;* Tam. *Kannakompu.*

A moderate or large tree; it is common in the dry and less common in the moist region of the low country of Ceylon, and also in South India and Malaya generally. Attygalle is of opinion that the Ceylon Ayurvedists mistakenly use *Myristica Horsefieldia,* the properties of which are quite different, for *Priyangu.*

It is said to be cooling and astringent and useful in febrile and inflammatory affections. It is also useful in the "burning" of the body and painful micturition. The seeds appear to be the part to which the medicinal reputation of the fruit is due. They are remarkably acid and astringent and when dry have an aromatic odour.. The fruit is sweet, astringent and tonic.

Amoora Rohituka, Hiern. Sinh. *Hingul;* Sans. *Rohituka, Rohini;* Tam. *Raktarohita.*

A moderate-sized evergreen tree, rather rare in the moist region of Ceylon. It is also found in Malabar, Bengal, Malaya, Andamans and the Phillipines.

It is regarded as a remedy for enlarged glands, spleen and liver and also against corpulence. It is considered to be of peculiar efficacy in enlarged spleen, hence the two Sanskrit names " plihaghna, spleen destroyer and " plihas tara," enemy of the spleen. The fruit is purgative and the bark astringent. In Bengal an oil is expressed from the seed; it is used for burning and as a stimulating liniment in rheumatism. The seeds are fried and bruised, then boiled with water when the oil floats on the surface.

The Pharm. Indica mentions that the bark contains two yellow resins soluble in ether, one of them insoluble in alcohol and alkaline solution, the other soluble in such liquids and of an acid nature. The alcoholic extract contains both soluble and insoluble tannin.

Azadirachta indica, Adr., or *Melia azadirachta, Linn.*, Eng, *Margosa or Indian lilac.* Sinh. *Kohomba;* Sans. *Ravipriya, Vimbaka, Vranashobakari;* Tam. *Vembu, Veppan.*

A large tree cultivated all over India on account of its medicinal properties. Every part of the plant is used in medicine. Generally, the tree is regarded as antiseptic, astringent and tonic and is given frequently in decoctions for fever. The astringent and antiseptic virtues of the bark have been experimentally confirmed. The seeds yield a very bitter oil which is an indispensable article in lying-in rooms. A dose of the oil is given internally to the mother after delivery of the child; it is applied to the parts and the room is fumigated daily with it. The bark and the leaves are largely used in the treatment of skin disease of every sort. The dried flowers are used as a tonic after fever and the medicine, *Pancha-nimba,* is a preparation consisting of the flowers, fruit, leaves, bark and root of the tree, of each 15 parts, and one part each of a number of other drugs.

It is also one of the five bitters, *Pancha-tikta.* The fruit is described as purgative, emollient and anthelmintic. The leaves are added to poultices to disperse glandular tumours and are used generally as a discutient; beaten into a pulp they are applied to pustular eruptions, more especially to the eruption of small-pox. The oil of the seeds is applied to suppurating scrofulous glands and is given in leprosy and rheumatism.

Neem or Margosa oil extracted from the seeds was examined by Warden (Pharm. Ind.). Its sp. gr. at 15.5° was 0.9235. It congealed at 10-7° without losing its transparency. It gave no characteristic colour reactions. It did not dry even when a thin film was exposed to a temperature of 100°. With alcohol there was extracted from it a very bitter substance, which possessed in a marked degreethe peculiar odour of the oil. The acids found were butyric, valeric, lauric, stearic and oleic.

The bark contains a bitter principle, which is a neutral resin. Broughton (Pharm. Journ. Trans. [3], iii, 992; Chem. Soc., 1873, 1157) isolated it by exhausting the bark with 60% alcohol and precipitating with water. The formula was obtained by making the nitro-derivative, $C_{36}H_{46}(NO_2)_4O_{11}$ giving $C_{36}H_{50}O_{11}$ for the resin. The leaves contain a small amount of a bitter substance of a similar nature, but far more soluble in water. This is a hydrate of the bitter principle of the bark.

The related tree, *Melia Toosendan*, Sieb. & Zucc. is of great value in domestic medicine in China. The fruits which are fleshy, globular drupes, are said to drive away infection and are employed as vermifuge and febrifuge. The root is also very bitter and is given for cutaneous diseases.

Melia Azedarach, Linn., Eng. *the Persian Lilac; the Indian Neem.* Sinh. *Lunumidella;* Sans. *Mahanimba;Hemadruma;* Tam. *Malai vempu.*

This is a large tree indigenous to India. The variety found in Ceylon is *Melia dubia,* Cav., which is rather common in the moist low country. Its wood is a cheap light timber. The leaves, fruit and bark are bitter in taste and have various medicinal properties. Within the fleshy portion of the fruit there is a bitter kernel from which "neem oil" is extracted by pressure.

The root bark is used in decoction as an anthelmintic for children. The leaf juice also has this property. The flowers and leaves applied as a poultice relieve nervous headaches. A decoction of the leaves is employed in hysteria. The leaves and bark are used internally and externally in leprosy. The root bark has been placed in the secondary list of U. S. Pharmacoepia as an anthelmintic. In large doses the drug produces narcotism followed by death.

Neem oil or Margosa oil was first examined by Harden (Pharm. Ind. i, p. 328) who found that the bitterness of the oil could be removed by repeated agitation with alcohol. By saponification he found butyric acid, a trace of valeric acid, and a snow-white acid, m.p., 43.6° which he described as lauric acid. No quantitative separation was made.

Chatterjie and Sen (Indian Medical Gazette, 1919, 54, 74) claimed to have isolated an acid of the linoleic acid series, in 23% yield, which they called margosic acid.

Watson, Mukherjee and Mukherjee (J. Soc. Chem. Ind. 1923, 42, 387T) isolated an amorphous bitter substance, $C_{15}H_{20}O_5$ and a crystalline bitter substance, margosopicrin $C_{24}H_{32}O_8$, a hydroxy acid. They challenge Chatterjee and Sen's formula (above) for margosic acid, which they think is $C_{18}H_{34}O_3$.

Roy and Dutt (J. Soc. Chem. Ind. 1929, 48, 333T) have investigated the oil. They find that Chatterjee & Sen's margosic acid is impure oleic acid and that the unsaponifiable matter contains a phytosterol. The acids present are lower fatty acids and stearic, palmitic, oleic, linoleic, arachidic and lignoceric acids and unsaturated resinous acids.

Munronia pumila, Sinh. *Binkohomba,*—is a very small shrub, common in rocky places in the low country of Ceylon. This must not be confounded with another plant which has the same Sinhalese name, and Sans. *Buminba,* which is *Ophelia chirata* or *Swetia chirata.*

Walsura piscida, Roxb. Sinh. *Kirikon, Molpetta;* Sans. *Walsura;* Tam. *Chadewakku,*—is a small or moderate sized tree, very common in the dry region of the low country of Ceylon; also in Malabar and Travancore.

The bark is regarded as a powerful, even dangerous, emmenagogue and also acts as a violent emetic. An ointment for itch is prepared with its fruit; it also kills vermin. It has been experimentally found to be stimulant and expectorant.

The bark is used in India to stupefy fish. This property has been experimentally verified and a further fact observed that fish killed with it still retains its wholesomeness as food.

RHAMNACEAE

Colubrina asiatica, Sinh. *Welheeriya;* Tam. *Mayirmanikkam,*—is a much-branched shrub, rather common an the dry region of Ceylon and also throughout India and Malaya and in Australia and S.W.Africa. It is istringent and is used in decoctions in which an astringent is required.

Rhamnus: Trimen records only two species of this genus:—*R.Arnottianus* and *R.Wightii.*

R.Arnottiana, is a small tree found in the upper montane zone of Ceylon, but rather rare.

R.Wightii, W. & A.,—is a large shrub, common in the upper montane of Ceylon. It is nearly allied to *R.Frangula,* the Alder-buckthorn of England. In India, R.*Wightii* is used in medicine as *Raktha-rohida,* the bark being highly esteemed for its tonic, astringent and deobstruent properties.

The bark has been examined by D.Hooper (Pharm. Journ., Feb. 1888), who found, among many other substances the following :—several resins, both reducing and non-reducing sugars, cathartic acid, malic acid, calcium oxalate, suberin, etc. (for a resume' see Pharm. Ind. i, 354)

Ventilago Madraspatana, Gaertn. Sinh. *Kobowakka or Yakadawel;* Sans. *Raktavalli;* Tam. *Vempafam, Suralpattai, Pappilichakkai.*

A large much-branched, woody climber, very common in the low country of Ceylon and in the plains of India.

The powdered root-bark is carminative, stomachic, tonic and stimulant. It is a powerful astringent and is used for tanning. Pounded with gingelly oil it is used as an application for itch. The bark of the stem serves as cordage.

Its root bark yields a dye, called *Popli,* which has been investigated by Perkin and Hummel (J. Chem. Soc. 1894, 65,923). Carbon disulphide extracts from the root bark five crystalline substances, which were separated by fractional crystallization, besides a wax and a resinous colouring matter. (1) $C_{16}H_{12}O_5$. which the authors regard as emodin mono-methyl ether, orange-red crystals melting at 200°. It yields a diacetyl derivative, m.p., 186° and a mono-nitro compound, m.p., 215-217°. When distilled with zinc dust a hydrocarbon melting at 203° is obtained (α -methyl anthracene). Its behaviour with zinc dust in alkaline solution shows it to be an α-methyl-anthraquinone derivative. It has one methoxy group.

(2) $C_{16}H_{14}O_4$, long colourless crystals, decomposing at 260°, yields a -methylanthracene and (probably) a triacetyl compound. Gentle oxidation with chromic acid or with alkaline hydrogen peroxide converts it to substance (1). Boiling fuming nitric acid converts it to a tetra-nitro compound. It is, therefore, trihydroxy-α-methyl-anthranole monomethyl ether.

(3) $C_{16}H_{14}O_4$, crystalllises in pale yellow needles, m.p., 173°, yields a tetra-acetylderivative, melting at 229°. It is probably trihydro xy α – methylanthranole monomethyl ether.

(4) $C_{16}H_8O_8$, orange-red crystalline powder, darkening at 260° and decomposing at 275-280°. It is sparingly soluble in most solvents. The yield was only 1% and the substance should be further examined.

(5) $C_{17}H_{12}O_5$, chocolate coloured crystalline substance.

The wax $(C_9H_{16}O)_n$ consists of nearly colourless-needles, m.p., 72°. The resinous colouring matter is a reddish-brown brittle resin $C_{15}H_{14}O_6$, m.p., 100-110°, and was impossible to crystallize.

As a dye the root bark presents no difficulty in its application. No additions to the dye-bath are necessary except in the cases of wool and silk, when it is advantageous to use a small percentage of copper acetate to correct the acidity of the mordanted fibre. On cotton, with aluminium mordant a purplish-red is obtained, while with iron mordant black to grey.

There are several species of the genus *Zizyphus* in Ceylon: *Zizyphus jujuba,* Lamk., and *Z.vulgaris,* Lam., Sinh. *Dabara* or *Masan* (Portuguese word) Sans. *Soubira.* The former is a small thorny spreading tree and is a native of Ceylon, India, Malaya, etc., found chiefly in the dry districts. The pulp of the fruit which is edible is rather pleasantly acid in flavour.

Z.vulgaris is a small thorny tree, native of Syria and the Levant. The dried fruits are regarded as expectorant and blood-purifier. A syrup useful in bronchitis is made out of them.

Z.Napeca, Sinh. *Yak-eraminiya;* Sans. *Kakoli,* is found in the low country, but rather rare. Since it is difficult to obtain, the Ayurvedists recommend the use of *Asvagandha* or *Satamula* as a substitute.

Z.Oenoplia, Mill., Sinh. *Heen-eraminiya,* is a scrambling shrub, very common in the low country, chiefly in the dry region. It is also found in Tropical Asia and Australia. The bark is used as a febrifuge and digestive tonic; it is also astringent and used in dysentery.

Z.rugosa, Lamk., Sinh. *Maha-eraminiya,* is a large straggling or climbing bush, common in the moist low country of Ceylon and in East Himalaya, Burma and South India. The flowers with an equal quantity of the petioles of the betel leaf and half as much lime are given in four grain pills twice a day for menorrhagia.

CELASTRACEAE

Celastrus paniculatus, Willd., Eng. *the Staff Tree,* Sinh, *Duhudu, Doodu;* Sans. *Jyotishmati, Kanguni, Vanhiructu. Katumbi;* Tam. *Atoparichcham.*

A large climbing shrub, in the moist low country of Ceylon and throughtout India, Malaya and the Philippines. The ripe fruit is a very pretty object and the seed is very often solitary.

The oil from the seeds is rubefacient. The seeds are alterative, stimulant and nervine.

The seeds yield by expression a deep scarlet or violet oil, which deposits a quantity of fat after it has been kept a short time. Its odour is pungent and acrid. It is much admired as an external application along with a poultice of the crushed seeds. On destructive distillation with benzoin, cloves, nutmegs and mace, the seeds yield " Oleum Nigrum ", a black, oily fluid employed in the treatment of beri-beri. In doses of ten to fifteen drops twice a day it acts as a powerful stimulant and generally produces free diaphoresis.

The seed oil applied to the head or the seeds given internally are supposed to strengthen the memory and thinking faculties. The oil is, therefore, used in some parts of India by students. The treatise " Jyotishmathi Kalpa " deals with the preparation and uses of this oil. The decoction of the seeds and the oil are also given in rheumatism, gout, paralysis and leprosy. The seed is sometimes administered by commencing with a dose of one seed and increasing by one daily, until thirty are taken and then for another thirty days, reducing the dose by one seed a day.

The leaf juice is given as an antidote to opium-smoking.

Elaeodendron glaucum, Pers. Sinh. *Neralu;* Sans. *Bhutapala;* Tam. *Pujari; Chellupaimaram.*

A small tree, common in the dry parts of Ceylon, especially near the coast and also in India & the Malay Archipelago; the leaves vary extremely.

The powdered leaves have a powerful sternutatory action and are used as a fumigatory to rouse women from hysterical syncope and as a snuff to relieve headache. The leaves rubbed into a paste are supposed to remove every sort of swelling. The root is regarded as an antidote to snake poison; experiments made by Dymock and others, however, show that there are no grounds for this belief.

The Sanskrit name means "Expeller of Demons," as hysteria is supposed to be caused by demons.

The bark contains an alkaloid separable by lime and chloroform. It gives a purplish colour with sulphuric acid and a yellow colour with nitric acid. Two resins have also been found, one of which is soluble in ether and warm amyl alcohol and the other in rectified spirit.

Kokuna zeylanica, Thw. Sinh. *Kokun;* Sans. *Kila, Kunkuma.*

This a very large tree rather rare in forests of the moist regions of Ceylon and South India.

The inner bark has a brilliant yellow colour. It is powdered, mixed with water, made into a paste, dried in the sun and formed into flat pieces largely used in place of soap. It has a pleasant smell and makes the skin smooth.

The oil of *K.zeylanica* is mentioned by Frederick Lewis as being much used by pilgrims to Adam's Peak (Ceylon) for protection against leeches.

Salacia prinoides, Sinh. *Heen-himbutuwel;* Sans. *Kushan*— is a large, climbing shrub, rather rare, found chiefly in the dry regions of Ceylon, and also in India, Malaya and the Philippines.

Salacia reiculata Sinh. *Himbutuwel, Kothala-himbutu,*— is a large, woody climber, rather common in the moist low country of Ceylon. It is very frequently used to allay thirst in cases of diabetes, for which purpose an infusion of the root is used. This drug should be investigated.

AMPELIDEAE

Leea macrophylla, Roxb., Sinh. *Burulla, Gurulla;* Sans. *Dholasamudrika.*

A large semi-shrubby annual, very common in the low country of Ceylon and throughtout the Eastern Tropics. It is a native of the hotter parts of India. The leaves when bruised have a pleasant scent, like apples; they turn black on drying.

In Ceylon the pulpy substance enclosed in the stem of the plant is fried in gingelly oil and applied to burns. The juice of the young leaves is digestive. The roasted leaves are applied to the head in vertigo. The tuberous root is employed in the cure of guinea worm and when pounded is applied to obstinate sores to promote cicatrization. It is astringent and is a reputed remedy in India for ringworm.

Vitis indica, Sinh. *To-wel, Rata-bulatwel;* Eng. *Indian wild vine.*

A shrub, common in the moist low country of Ceylon and in Western Peninsular India. The fruit very much resembles that of the grape vine, *V.vinifera,* but is bitter in taste.

In decoction it is alterative and is considered to render the secretion healthy. The root juice mixed with oil is an application in eye diseases. Combined with coconut milk it is applied to carbuncles and other malignant ulcers.

Vitis quandrangularis, Sinh. *Heeressa, Seeressa ;* Sans. *Ashtisandhana, Vajravalli;* Tam. *Pirandai.*
This is very common in the dry regions of Ceylon and also in India, Malaya, Java and Tropical Africa.

The young leaves and tender shoots are eaten as a vegetable. When old they become acrid and seem to possess medicinal properties; they are dried, powdered and given in certain bowel complaints connected with indigestion and are also considered powerful alteratives. The juice of the stem is dropped into the ear for otorrhoea and into the nose in epistaxis. It has also a reputation in scurvy and irregular menstruation. It is an ingredient, along with opium, in a confection for dysentery.

Vitia vinifera, Eng. *the grape vine;* Sinh. *Mudrappalam;* Tam. *Diraksha Pazham,*—is not a native of Ceylon. The dried fruit, raisin, has been used in Ayurveda for a long time. It is given in combination with other drugs and is an ingredient in several ghritas, churnas, confections, etc.

The mucilage of *V.pentapylla* contains araban and galactan. (Abst. 1896, i, 61). Petri (Abst., 1911, ii, 325) states that the roots of many kinds of vine contain a substance which gives a blue colouration with ferric chloride. The substance can be extracted with alcohol at 70-80°. Power & Chestnut (J. Am. Chem. Soc. 1921, 43, 1741) have found methyl anthranilate in grape juice.

SAPINDACEAE

Allophylus Cobbe, Sinh. *Kobo, Bookobo;* Sans. *Kapolawattha;* Tam. *Amarai,*—is a tall much-branched shrub, very common in the low country of Ceylon, particularly in the moist region. The Veddahs employ the wood for making bows. The little pulpy fruit is eaten.

It is tonic, alexipharmic and emmenagogue. Fumigations with this are useful in hysteria. Mixed with scammony it makes a good purgative.

Allophylus zeylanicus, Sinh. *Wal-kobo,*—is a small tree or shrub, rather common in the moist region.

Cardiospermum Halicacabum, Linn, Eng. *Balloon Vine or Winter Cherry;* Sinh. *Penelawel;* Sans. *Jyotishmati, Paravata-padi, (Pigeon's Foot), Lataphatki;* Tam. *Mudukottan.*

It is an annual herb, which is very common in the low country of Ceylon and throughout the Tropics.

It is very largely used by the Sinhalese bone-setters to allay pains in sprains and contusions about the joints. In decoction the roots and the leaves are used in rheumatism, nervous diseases, haemorrhoids, chronic bronchitis and phthsis. The juice of the leaves is dropped into the ears for earache. The leaves are used in amenorrhoea. A compound powder made of potassium carbonate, the root of *Acorus Calanus* (*Vada-kaha*), root bark of *Terminalia tomentosa* (*heen-kumbuk*) is recommended in the medical work, " Bhavaprakasha " for amenorrhoea.

The Pharm. Indica states that the properties of this plant are due to the presence of saponin.

Nephelium longana, Camb. Eng. *Longan tree or Dragon's eye;* Sinh. *Mora, Rasamora;* Sans. *Pilu;* Tam. *Nurai.*

A large tree common in the low country of Ceylon and in South India, East Bengal, Burma and South China. The wood is moderately hard and heavy. The aril of the seed is edible and very sweet, but is inferior to that of *N.lappaceum.* The aril is used as a refrigerant in fevers. The leaves and flowers of the longan tree are officinal in China but, possibly, only from recent times.

Nephelium lappaceum, Linn., Sinh. *Rambutan*,—is a large handsome spreading tree, a native of Malaya. It was introduced into Ceylon but curiously enough is little known in India, Mauritius, Madagascar, etc. It is, however, not used in medicine in Ceylon. In Malaya, decoction of the bark is used in diseases of the tongue.

Its seeds have been examined by Baczewski (Monatsh. 1895, 16, 866; Ber., 1896, 29 R, 30). He found that on the average the seeds contain 5.87% water, 35% oil, 25.6% starch, 1.25% sugar. The oil gave the following values :—m.p. 42-46°, solidifies at 38-39°. sp. gr., 0.9236, acid value 42.9, saponification value 193.8, Reichert-Meissl value 2.2, Iodine value 39.4. The acids present are :—Arachic, oleic and traces of stearic.

Sapindus trifoliatus, Linn., Eng. *Soap nut tree;* Sinh. *Penela;* Sans. *Arishta, Penila;* Tam. *Neykkoddan, Panalai, Poovandi.*

A large tree, common in the forests of the dry region of Ceylon and also throughout India and Burma.

It has been long used as a detergent, hence the English name. Medicinally it is regarded as hot and alexipharmic. Four grains in wine cure colic. The pulp is, in small doses, anthelmintic and is also given in cases of snake bites. It is given in severe diarrhoea and cholera for which the pulp is rubbed into water until it soaks, strained and given by the mouth.

Paranjpe and Ayyar (J. Indian Inst. Sci. 1929, 12A, 179) have investigated the chemistry of the fruits and seeds of this tree. The fruits are fleshy, two or three united, and each is the size of a cherry. The seeds resemble the fruit in shape. The fruits contain 65.7% pericarp and 34.3% seed. The finely powdered seed kernels gave, on extraction with ligroin, 44.7% of a dark yellow oil, which deposits, a small quantity of stearin on standing. The remarkable property of this oil is that it contains 22% of the glyceride of n-eicosoic acid, other acids present are palmitic stearic, oleic and lignoceric. It may be classed as a non-drying oil, the iodine value being 58.5. In 1910 Menon (J. Soc. Chem. Ind. 1910, 1431) had also investigated this oil and obtained the values given below.

	P. & A.	Menon
Sp.gr. 100/100°	0.8540	0.8542
$n_D^{25°}$	1.4764	1.4748
Sap. Value	194.1	191.8
Reichert-Meissl value	1.5	1.6
Unsap. matter	1.2%	1.1%
Iodine value	58.5	58.6

Sapindus laurifolu, Sinh. *Kaha-penala,* has similar uses.

Sapindus mukrossi, Gaertn., is the soap nut tree of China and Japan (not found in Ceylon). The fruits are used as soap and contain 10% saponin. The round, hard, brown seeds are called Bodhi seeds because they are made into necklaces and worn by Buddhists as rosaries. The solution of the fruits is a remedy for cutaneous diseases.

The following species (not found in Ceylon) have been investigated :—*Sapindus Rarak,* has been examined by May (Arch. Pharm., 1906, *244,* 25; Abst., 1906, ii, 301). He isolated from the powdered husks, in 13.5% yield, a saponin $C_{24}H_{42}O_{15}$, which when heated with 5% HCl or H_2SO_4 gave a sapogenin $C_{12}H_{18}O_3$, a pentose and a hexose. The embryo freed from husk gave 26.2% of a yellow non-drying oil, Sp. gr., 0.911 at 15°, acid value 5.3, sap. value 170.2, iodine value 65.1, Reichert-Meissl value 0.7 The acids present are oleic 80%, palmitic 16%, and stearic 4%.

Asahina and Shimidzu (Abst., 1916, i, 734) obtained from *S.mukrossi* a saponin as an amorphous white powder $[\alpha]_D^{20°}$ + 13.28, which on hydrolysis gave d-arabinose and a sapogenin.

Winterstein (Z physiol. Chem, 1919, 104, 217; Abst., 1919, i, 373) isolated sucrose from *S.utilis.*

Schleichera trijuga, Willd., Eng. *the Ceylon Oak;* Sinh. *Kon;* Sans. *Pilu;* Tam. *Pumaram.*

A large slow-growing tree of Ceylon, India, Burma, etc. It takes 16-18 years to grow to a sufficient size before it can yield heavy crops of superior lac every second or third year. The tree is the *Kusum* or *Kusumb* of India.

The pulpy aril is acid. The bark is astringent and mixed with oil it is an external application for itch.

The oil, which is used as a lamp oil in India, is reputed to be the original Macassar oil. It was re-introduced into Germany as Macassar oil and has been noticed as a valuable stimulating and cleansing application to the scalp, promoting the growth of hair.

ANACARDIACEAE

Anacardium occidentale, Linn., Eng. *Cashew nut;* Sinh. *Kaju;* Sans. *Kajutaka, Shoephara;* Tam. *Mundiri-maram, Kottai-mundari.*

This tree is so completely established in the low country of Ceylon, especially on sandy ground near the sea, as to have all the look of a native tree. It was introduced from Brazil by the Portuguese; it was therefore not known to the old Sanskrit writers.

The oil or tar obtained from the pericarp is an effective preventive against insects. The edible fruit is a remedy for scurvy. The nut gives about 47% of an oil having the following properties :—sap. value 195, Iod. val. 84, $[\alpha]_D^{20°}$ 1.4702.

Buchanania latifolia, Roxb., Cheronjee; Sans. *Piyala, Chara Chirka Tapasapriya;* Tam. *Katma.*

A small tree native of the mountainous parts of Coromandel, Malabar, Mysore, etc., The pear-shaped kernels of the fruits are sometimes used as a substitute for almonds and a fine oil, known as Cheronjee Oil, is expressed from them. The fruit, seed, gum, root and leaves are used in medicine in India. The tree is not known in Ceylon, but a close ally, *B.augustifolia, Roxb.*, is indigenous. It grows best in the low country but is rather rare. The fruit does not appear to be eaten.

In India, the seeds of *B.latifolia* are an article of commerce and are used in the preparation of sweetmeats. The seeds have been examined by Chirch (Pharm. Ind.). The expressed oil congeals at 18.5°, at which temperature its sp. gr. is 0.9134. It gives 95% of fatty acids which contain oleic, stearic and palmitic acids.

Mangifera indica, Linn., Eng, *Mango tree;* Sinh. *Amba;* Sans. *Amra, Chuta,* Tam. *Mankai.*

This tree is indigenous to India and has been cultivated from time immemorial for the fruit, *the* fruit par excellence, of India. The variety indigenous to Ceylon is *M.zeylanica,* Sinh. *Atamba.*

The ripe fruit is laxative and diuretic and useful in in nervous and atonic dyspepsia; when unripe the fruit is astringent.

The powdered seed has been recommended as an anthelmintic (for lumbrici) in doses of 20-30 grains and also as an astringent in bleeding piles and menorrhagia. The seed kernel is used as an astringent in decoctions for dysentery.

The unripe fruit contains tartaric acid with a trace of citric acid. The orange colouring matter of the ripe fruit is a chlorophyll product, readily soluble in ether, carbon disulphide and benzene, but less readily in benzene.

Odina Wodier, Roxb., vel Rhus odina, Sinh. *Hik;* Sans. *Jingini, Ajashringi;* Tam. *Odiya-maram.*

A small deciduous tree, common in the low country of Ceylon, especially in the dry region, and throughout India, Burma, and the Andaman Islands. It is one of the few deciduous trees of Ceylon. The heartwood is red, rather heavy, moderately hard and close-grained and is used for timber.

The bark is used as a collyrium for sore eyes. The powdered bark and margosa oil make a useful application for old and incurable ulcers. The decoction of the bark has been recommended as an astringent gargle.

The tree exudes a gum which, beaten up with coconut milk, is applied to sprains and bruises and the leaves boiled in oil are used for the same puropse.

Semecarpus anacardium, Linn., Eng. *Marking nut tree;* Sinh. *Senkottan;* Sans. *Bhallataka, Agnimukhi, Arushkara;* Tam. *Shenkottai.*

This tree grows on the mountainous parts of Tropical India but not in Ceylon. The kernel of the nut contains a small quantity of sweet oil. The acrid juice of the nut leaves an indelible stain on cotton. It was also used in the old days in medicine as a vesicant. In combination with other drugs it is given in various diseases, such as dyspepsia, leprosy, skin diseases and nervous disorders. A powerful restorative, *Amrita Bhallataka,* is recommended by Chakradatta, and is made as follows :—Ripe marking nuts divided into halves, 8 seers, boil in 20 seers water down to 5 seers and strain. Again boil the nuts in 16 seers of milk and 4 of clarified butter to a thick consistence. Add 2 seers of sugar and set aside for 7 days. Dose 20-90 grains twice a day with milk.

In the Concan, a single fruit is heated in the flame of a lamp and the oil allowed to drop into a quarter seer of milk, and this is given daily in cough caused by relaxation of the uvula and palate. The brown oil of the marking nut appears to resemble that of the cashew nut in its medicinal action. The nut is used in India as a local irritant to procure abortion. (Pharm. Ind.).

Semecarpus coriacea, S.Gardnei, S.obscura (Sinh. *Badulla;* Sans. *Bhallataka*), *S.obvota* (Sinh. *Kalu-badulla*), *S.subpellata* (Sinh. *Maha-badulla*) are similar to *S.anacardium* in properties and uses.

Spondias mangifera, Willd., Wild mango, Sinh. *Ambrella;* Sans. *Amrataka;* Tam. *Ampallai, Marimanchedi,*—is a small moderate sized tree, common in the moist low country of Ceylon and throughout Tropical Asia.

The pulp of the fruit is astringent and is useful in dyspepsia and is on that account called *Pitha-vriksha,* Bile tree. It is made into pickles and preserves. The gum exuding from the tree is used in fumigation.

COMBRETACEAE

Anogeissus latifolia, Wall., Sinh. *Dava;* Sans. *Dhavala, Madhura-tvacha, Vakavriksha;* Tam. *Vekkali.*

A small tree growing on open grass lands in the dry region of Ceylon (rare, but locally abundant) and also in Peninsular India. The fruit resembles the head of a crane, hence the last Sanskrit name, which means " Crane-tree."

The decoction of the leaves is given in diarrhoea and gonorrhoea. The gum collected from the flowers is used as a substitute for gum-arabic and gum acacia and is also used by Indian calico printers as a mordant for fixing colours.

The leaves contain 15% tannic acid.

Terminalia arjuna, Bedd., vel Terminalia glabra, W & A.. Sinh. *Kumbuk;* Sans. *Arjuna;* Tam. *Vellai-maruda-maram,*

A very large tree with an extremely thick trunk and horizontally spreading branches, rare in the moist districts but very common in the dry regions of Ceylon and India.

In action the bark is astringent, cardiac stimulant, tonic and lithontriptic. It is used internally in dysentery, fever and heart diseases. With milk, treacle or water it is given in fractures and contusions with extensive ecchymosis, as it is said to promote union of fractures. Charaka recommends the powdered bark and an equal quantity of red sandalwood with sugar and rice water for haemoptysis. Externally the leaves are used for covering ulcers and sores. The bark well-pounded with goat's milk is given to stop bleeding in dysentery.

The ash contains an "immense" quantity of lime. There is a belief among the Sinhalese that a "kumbuk" tree close to a well improves its water. This is probably due to the large absorption of lime by the roots. The ash of the bark is used for chewing with betel.

Terminalia bellerica, Roxb., Beleric myrobalans; Sinh. *Bulu;* Sans. *Vibhitaka (fearless), Anilaghnaka (wind-killing)* Tam. *Tanti.*

A large tree with straight and long horizontal branches; growing in the low country of Ceylon (but not common) and in India and Malaya.

The properties and uses of this are nearly the same as those of *aralu* (*T.chebula, q.v.*). It is an ingredient in many decoctions and other preparations for various diseases. It is a constituent of the Sanskrit "Triphala," Sinhalese "Tipala," which consists of chebulic, beleric and emblic myrobalans. A very efficacious preparation for sore eyes of all sorts is composed of long pepper, black pepper, margosa leaves and chebulic and beleric myrobalans reduced to a fine paste with cow's urine, made into pellets and dried in the shade; the addition of a little orpiment and chalk improves the keeping power of the preparation.

The kernel is said to be narcotic and astringent and is used as an application to inflamed parts. An oil expressed from the kernel is used as a dressing for the hair and as a substitute for ghee.

Terminalia Catappa, L., Country or Indian almond, Sinh. *Kottamba;* Tam. *Kottai.*

This is a medium sized or large tree with large handsome shining leaves, native of Malaya but now grown in most tropical countries. It drops its leaves twice a year (Feb. & Sept. in Ceylon). The Sinhalese name is a corruption of the Malaya "catappa."

The kernel is edible and is similar to the almond except in size. The bark is astringent and yields a black pigment used by some in India to colour the teeth. The leaves contain tannin. The juice of the young leaves is employed to prepare an ointment for scabies, leprosy and other cutaneous diseases. The kernels yield 50% of an oil resembling almond oil for which it is used as a substitute.

Terminalia chebula, Retz., (Chebulic or black myrobalans,) Eng. *Ink nuts, Gall nuts;* Sinh. *Aralu;* Sans. *Haritaki;* Tam. *Kadukkai.*

A moderate sized deciduous tree of Ceylon, India and Burma. The flesh of the fruit is rich in tannin and the dried ovoid fruits (nuts) are used largely in dyeing and tanning.

Besides being an ingredient in the "Triphala," it enters into many preparations. It is regarded as tonic, alterative and laxative. As a laxative it is given both singly and in combination with other drugs. In action it is very much like rhubarb in that it first acts as purgative followed by confinement of the bowels. Roasting or baking the nuts prevents the laxative action; prepared in this way it is given in cases of dysentery in all its stages. In young king coconut water it also acts as a mild cathartic. A collyrium prepared with it and alum is useful for sore eyes; according to Attygalle this is superior to zinc lotion.

Terminalia tomentosa, W & A., Sinh. & Sans. *Asana;* Tam. *Matura-maram,*—is met with in the Deccan. According to Trimen, this species is very doubtfully distinct from *T.glabra.*

The fixed oils derived from the *Genus Terminalia* have the following properties :—

	Yield	Sap. val.	Iod.Val.	Sp.gr.
T.Catappa	30.0	190.5	91.8	—
T.Belerica	48.3	203-204	81.8	0.9206
T.Chebula	25.0	205.8-205.3	79-95	0.9168-0.9193

(Lewkowitsch, ii, 484)

Friedolin (Chem. Zentr. 1884, 641; Abst. 1885, 396) isolated from the fruit of *T.chebula* an acid which he called chebulinic acid. Its percentage composition approaches that of gallic acid, which it resembles in some properties but differs in others. It is soluble in alcohol and hot water, but sparingly in cold.

Perkin (J. Chem. Soc., 1897,71, 1137) has examined *T.chebula.* It contains no quercetin or allied series but contains ellagic and ellagitannic acids, the presence of which were also confirmed by it's dyeing properties.

MYRTACEAE

Barringtonia acutangula, Gaertn., Ela-midella; Sans. *Hijjala;* Tam. *Kadapum,.*

A small tree with thick trunk and brownish grey bark, found in the dry region round margins of tanks and similar places in Ceylon and throughout India, being plentiful in Bengal. It also grows in Malaya and Australia.

The seed is aromatic, carminative and emetic. The bitter root is similar to cinchona in properties. The powdered seeds are used as snuff. In general, the properties are the same as those of *B.racemosa* (see below).

Barringtonia racemosa, Blume, Sinh. *Diya-midella;* Sans. *Vishaya, etc.,* is a small tree with long drooping branches. It is common in the moist low country of Ceylon; it flowers (slightly scented) all the year round. It also grows on the Malabar coast and in Malaya and Polynesia.

The root is similar to cinchona in medicinal properties and is deobstruent and cooling. The fruit is spoken of as *Samudraphala* and *Dhatri-phala* or "nurse's fruit" and is one of the best known domestic remedies in India. When children suffer from a cold in the chest, the seed is rubbed down on a stone with water and applied over the sternum, and if there is much dyspnoea a few grains with or without the juice of fresh ginger are administered internally, and seldom fail to induce vomiting and the explusion of mucus from the air passages. (Pharm. Ind.). Two or three grains of the powdered seed are given in milk to reduce enlarged abdomen in children.

The active principle of the seeds of these two species seems to be a body allied to saponin. The aqueous solution forms a stable froth when shaken, and at first tastes sweet and afterwards bitter and acrid.

Barringtonia zeylanica, Sinh. *Goda-midella,* is a species indigenous to Ceylon and used as above in medicine.

Careya arborea, Roxb., Patana Oak, Sinh. *Kahata;* Sans. *Kumbhi;* Tam. *Kachaddai, Patai-tanni-maram* (*water-bark-tree*), on account of the exudation trickling down the bark in dry weather.

A small or middle-sized, deciduous tree, with very thick, rough, dark grey bark. It is very common, especially on exposed patana land and grows in the moist region of Ceylon up to 5000 ft. and also in sub-Himalayan India.

The bark is very astringent (hence the Sinhalese name) and is used in dysentery and fever accompanied with loose bowels. In snake bite the bark is applied to the wound and an infusion of it given internally. The leaves made into a poultice rapidly heal obstinate ulcers. The bark of the tree and the calices of the flowers are well-known Indian remedies and are valued on account of their astringent and mucilaginous properties, being administered in cough and applied externally as an embrocation. An astringent gum exudes from the fruit, and stem; the bark is made into coarse cordage.

Caryophyllus aromaticus, L., vel Eugenia caryophyllata, Thunb., Eng. *Cloves,* Sinh. *Karabu;* Sans. *Lavanga;* Tam. *Karuvappu.*

This tree is said to be indigenous only on Moluccas proper. It was afterwards introduced into other neighbouring islands, where it is now cultivated, and at a later period into Zanzibar and Pemba on the east coast of Africa. Cloves appear to have been known to China as early as B.C. 266. (Pharmacographia). It is difficult to say when they were introduced into India and Ceylon but Charaka mentions them under the name *Lavanga.*

They are regarded carminative, stomachic and stimulant and are used in many diseases in combination with other drugs. A clove roasted in the flame of a lamp and held in the mouth is a popular remedy for sore throat. A paste of cloves is applied to the forehead and nose as a remedy for colds. Mohamedan writers consider them to be alexipharmic and cephalic, whether taken externally or internally. They also recommend them for strengthening the gums. In modern medicine cloves are used as carminative and stimulant, to relieve irritation of the throat accompanied by racking cough, and to deaden the pain of toothache.

Eugenol is the most characteristic constituent of the essential oil ; other important constituents are aceteugenol, α–and β–caryophyllene. (For details see Gildemeister & Hoffmann, Volatile Oils or other work on Essential Oils).

Eugenia Corymbosa, Lam., Sinh. *Dan, Heen-dan;* Sans. *Svetha-jambu;* Tam. *Marungi.*

A bush or shrubby tree, very common especially in open sandy places in the low country of Ceylon and also in South India and Burma. The small black fruit is edible. The plant is only occasionally, if ever, used in medicine. Its properties are the same as those of *Eugenia jambolana.*

Eugenia jambolana, Lam., Sinh. *Maha-dan or Madan;* Sans. *Jambu, Rajaphala, Meghavarna;* Tam. *Naval, Perunaval.*

A large or very large tree, found in the low country of Ceylon and throughout Tropical Asia. Varieties with much larger fruits than the Ceylon fruit are found in India.

The sub-acid fruits are edible. Graeser has observed that the formation of sugar in dogs when phloridzin was administered for some time, was arrested when an extract of *Jambolanum* was given to the animals at the same time. It may, therefore, prove useful in diabetes melitus. Whether the active principle is contained in the pericarp or kernel has not been ascertained.

In 1889 Laveine obtained negative results with the seeds in three cases in which the urine contained 6 to 7% of sugar. In these cases powdered seeds were given in doses of one gram 4 to 6 times a day.

The bark, leaves and seeds are astringent. The bark, alone or with other astringents, is used in chronic diarrhoea and dysentery and as a gargle in sore throat. A vinegar prepared from the juice of the ripe fruit is an agreeable stomachic and carminative; it is also diuretic. A sort of spirituous liquor, called Jambava, is described in recent Sanskrit works as prepared by distilling the juice. The juice of the leaves is said to dissolve iron filings.

Eugenia jambu, L., the Jambu or Rose-apple,—is a Malayan species. The fruits are pleasantly sub-acid and refreshing.

Eugenia zeylanica var spicata,—is a Ceylon species, Sinh. *Maranda;* Tam. *Marungi.*

Psidium Guyava, Linn., Sinh. *Pera;* Tam. *Shivappu-goyya-pazham or Vellai-goyya-pazham.*

A large spreading shrub or small tree, native of Tropical America. It was probably introduced into Ceylon by the Portuguese; in fact, the Sinhalese name is the Portuguese for pear. The fruits, which are pale yellow when ripe, are edible. They have numerous seeds and are used in making " guava jelly."

The seeds are injurious. The ripe fruit is a good aperient when eaten with the rind, but without the rind, it is said to cause costiveness. The unripe fruit is employed in the treatment of diarrhoea, as is the bark. A decoction of half an ounce of the root bark with six of water, boiled down to three ounces, is recommended by Waitz as a remedy for chronic diarrhoea of children. The same preparation is recommended as an external application in the prolapsus ani of children. A decoction of the young leaves and shoots is prescribed in the West Indies in febrifuge and antispasmodic baths, an infusion of the leaves in cerebral affections, nephritis and cachexia; the pounded leaves are locally applied in rheumatism; an extract is used in epilepsy and chorea; the tincture is rubbed into the spine of children suffering from convulsions. (Pharm. Ind.)

Altan (Abst., i, 265) has investigated the leaves and found :—3.15% resin, 5.99% fat, etc. The citron-yellow aromatic resin is readily soluble in chloroform, ether or alcohol; it melts at 189°, has Iod. Number 115, acid number 89, sap. number 131.

The volatile oil contains eugenol and boils at 237°, sp. gr. 1.069.

FICOIDEAE

Gisekia pharmacoides, L., Sinh. *Attirillpala;* Sans. *Valuka;* Tam. *Manal-kirai.*

A rather succulent herb, rather common in damp, sandy places in the low country of Ceylon and also in the drier parts of India, Afghanistan and Africa.

It is regarded as aromatic, anthelmintic and aperient and is used as a vegetable. A draught made by grinding the plant with its leaves, stalks, etc. is given in taenia; a dose of two ounces is given in the morning on an empty stomach and repeated three times at intervals of four days.

According to the authors of Pharm. Ind., the most important principles in the seeds are astringent principles, which they provisionally call α–and β–Gisekia tannin. The α–tannin is obtained by agitating an alcoholic extract with ether; it forms an orange varnish, in which nodules gradually form on standing, which on microscopic examination are seen to consist of narrow plates and a few needles of a deep yellow colour. β–Gisekia tannin occurs as a deep orange powder, and is obtained by acidulating the aqueous alcoholic extract after agitation with ether, when the tannin is precipitated. No alkaloid was detected and the anthelmintic properties of the seeds are considered to be due to the tannins.

Mollugo cerviana, Ser., (also *M.spergula* and *M.stricta*), Sinh. *Udetta;* Sans. *Phanija, Grishma-sundaraka;* Tam. *Patpadakam.*

An annual with very numerous and slender stems, rather common in the dry region of Ceylon, India and the rest of Asia, Africa and Australia.

M.spergula and *M.stricta* are varieties; all of them are considered stomachic, aperient and antiseptic and are used to suppress lochia; when applied warm and moistened with a little castor oil, it is reckoned a good application for ear-ache. Oil in which the plant is boiled is used as an application for gouty and rheumatic complaints.

M.stricta contains a bitter principle, soluble in ether, alcohol and water. Rectified spirit dissolves a bitter resin.

Trianthema decandra, L., Sinh. *Mahasarana;* Tam. *Charanai.*

A herb with long, prostrate branches, found chiefly in the dry region of the low country of Ceylon, but rather rare. It is also found in India and Burma. It has pretty flowers and its properties are the same as of *T.monogyna.*

Trianthema Monogyna, L., Sinh. *Heen-sarana;* Sans. *Sveta, Punarnava;* Tam. *Charanai.*

A prostrate, somewhat succulent herb, found throughout the Tropics, and in Ceylon on the coast and in the dry region.

It is regarded as diuretic, cathartic and emmenagogue. The root when fresh is sweet; dried and powdered, it is given with ginger as cathartic. An infusion of it is given in constipation, jaundice, strangury and dropsy; also in torpid liver, asthma and amenorrhoea. Young plants when well boiled are eaten as a vegetable. The herb is said to be an irritant to the uterus and is said to cause abortion.

The mucilaginous decoction of the plant is unaffected by idoine solution but is precipitated by ferric chloride and neutral lead acetate solutions. It gives a precipitate with barium hydroxide, which contains a glucoside having similar properties to saponin.

CORNACEAE

Alangium Lamarckii, Thw., Eng. *Sage-leaved Alangium;* Sinh. *Alanga;* Sans. *Ankotam Nicochaka, Gupta-sneha* (" the oil which is hidden"); Tam. *Alangai, Azhinji-maram.*

An erect tree of small size, rather common in Ceylon (dry and intermediate regions) and throughout India and Malaya, S. China, the Phillipines and East Africa.

It is demulcent, bitter, pungent and aperient. It expels worms, poisons, phelgm and wind. The root bark is emetic in doses of 50 grains; in smaller doses (10 grains), it is nauseant and febrifuge. Rubbed in rice water, it is given with a little honey in diabetes. The very bitter bark is used in skin diseases, leprosy and syphillis. It is a good substitute for *ipecacuanha,* except in cases of dysentery, and is called *Indian Ipecacuanha.* It is supposed to be one of the ingredients of the secret remedies used by specialists in the treatment of snake and mad dog bites.

"The most interesting principle present in the roots is a very bitter non-crystallizable alkaloid, which we have provisionally called Alangine. It is soluble in alcohol, ether, chloroform and acetic ether, and practically insoluble in water. A platinum salt was prepared which contained 20.703% of platinum in the salt dried at 100° (Pharm. Ind., ii, 166).

UMBELLIFERAE

Bupleurum virgatum, W & A, Sinh. *Wal-endaru,* is the only species of *Bupleurum* mentioned by Trimen. It is not used in medicine nor has its essential oil been investigated. It is an annual or perennial growing on the rocky, open places in the montane region of Ceylon, common on the eastern slopes but scarcely on the western.

The oil of *B.fructosium.* L., which grows abundantly in Sardinia, has been investigated. There is an increase of oil content during the development of the plant and the flowers contain more oil than the leaves; yield of oil from leaves is 1-3%, from the flowers 3.75% and from the entire plant 0.5 to 4.4%. Besides an alcohol and an ester, the oil contains a large amount of a terpene which resembles limonene and has the following properties :— b.p., 167-169°; sp.gr. at 14°, 0.8416; $[\alpha]_D{}^{17°}$ 35.7°; n, 1.4862;

polymerises at 200° to an amorphous white mass. The alcohol has been called Bupleurol and is regarded as an aliphatic alcohol of the formula,

$$\begin{array}{l} CH_3 \\ \quad > CH.CH_2.\ CH_2.\ CH_2.\ \underset{\underset{CH_2.}{\|}}{CH}\ CH_2\ OH. \\ CH_3 \end{array}$$

For details and literature, see Gildemeister & Hoffmann, Volatile Oils iii, 311 et seq.

Carum Carui, Linn. Eng. *Black cumin,* Sinh. *Kalu-duru;* Sans. *Sushava;* Tam. *Pilappu-shiragam.*

A kind of caraway, found in Kashmir, Gurwal and Persia. This appears to have been known to the Hindus before the introduction of European caraway. The seeds are described as aromatic, carminative and astringent. An eyewash prepared from them is supposed to strengthen the sight. They are also used as a pectoral, and considered to be diuretic and anthelmintic. A caraway bath is recommended for painful swellings of the womb, and a poultice for painful and protruding piles.

The chief constituents of the essential obtained from the seeds are carvene and carvol.

Carum Roxburghianum, Benth., (*Ptychotis Ajowan, D.C.*) Sinh. *Asamodagan;* Sans. *Yavanika, Ugraghanda* etc., Tam. *Omum.*

It is cultivated in gardens and is occasionally found as a weed. It is frequently used in domestic medicine as a carminative. The seeds are useful in flatulence, colic, atonic dyspepsia and spasmodic affections of the bowels. A very popular domestic remedy for diarrhoea in children is an infusion of the powder made by roasting the seeds of *C.Roxburghianum* and *Hola rhena antidysenterica* (Sinh. *Kelinda*). The root is regarded as diuretic and prescribed for anasarca. The plant was not used by ancient Hindu physicians but later by Arabian physicians.

The volatile oil is useful in the early stages of cholera to check the vomitting and purging.

Oil of Parsley is the essential oil obtained from *Carum Petroselinum* (Benth. et Hook), indigenous to the Mediterr-anean countries and to Central Asia but now cultivated in all temperate countries. The principal constituent of the German oil is apiol. The French oil gives pinene and traces of palmitic acid and phenols and ketones, not characterized. See Gildemister & Hoffmann, Volatile Oils iii, 523.

Hydrocotyle Asiatica, L., the Indian Pennywort, Sinh. *Heen-getakola;* Sans. *Brahmi or Mandukaparni;* Tam. *Vellarai.*

A very common weed in waste grassy places from sea-level to higher elevations in all tropical countries.

Hydrocotyle javanica, Thunb., Sinh. *Maha-getakola;* Sans. & Tam. names the same as above,—is common in moist places, in grass under trees, up to 7000 feet, in Ceylon, India, Malaya, Tropical Australia, and Tropical E. Africa.

These two plants are alterative, tonic, diuretic and local stimulant, especially of the cutaneous system. They have a special influence on the genito-urinary tract and set up urinary and ovarian irritation. Experiments carried out in Madras have shown that their reputation as specifics for leprosy is unfounded, although they were found to be most useful in ameliorating the symptoms and improving the general health.

H. asiatica was made officinal in the Pharmocopoeia of India and is described as alterative, tonic and local stimulant, more especially useful in syphilitic skin diseases, in which it may be used both as an internal and local remedy. The plant is more abundant in Mauritius, where it serves as forage for cattle, whose milk it improves. de Grandpre states that the plant should be very carefully dried and bottled so as to preserve the volatile oil which is the active principle, and that the whole plant should be used as he finds it more active than the leaves. In Malaya, it is used as a cooling medicine and tonic and for rheumatism and skin complaints.

Lepine (J. pharm. Chim., 3, xxviii, 46) found in it a peculiar body, which he named Vellarin, in 0.8 to 1.0% yield. It is an oily non-volatile liquid. Dymock and others could not, however, isolate this substance.

Peucedanum graveolens, Benth., Eng. *The Dill plant*, Sinh. *Satakuppa;* Sans. *Misreya, Satapushpa;* Tam. *Satakuppi-kirai.*

A biennial of Southern Europe, the aromatic leaves of which are used in soups, etc. The seeds yield an oil of medicinal value from which the well-known dill water is made. The plant is easily cultivated and thrives in various parts of India. It is used both as a condiment and as a medicine. It is usually given to women after confinement to promote the discharge of lochia and relieve after-pains.

Peucedanin or imperatorin,

$$CH_8O . C_6H_4 . O . C_6H_4 . O . CH_2 . CO . CH_3 \text{ (?)}$$

was isolated by Schlatter (Ann., *5*, 201) and Rothe (Jahresber., 1849, 475) from the roots of *P.officinale* and by Wackenroder and Wagner (Jahresber. 1854, 638) from the roots of *Imperatoria Ostruthium* by digesting with 90% alcohol for six days and diluting the solution; the solid crystallized from ether and ligroin in prisms, m.p., 76°. It gave a mono-nitro-derivative with cold nitric acid of specific gravity 1.3.

Jassoy and Haensel (Arch. der Pharm., *236*, 668) and Popper (Monatsh. *19*, 268) extracted peucedanin from *P.officinale* with a large quantity of warm ether and by purification obtained colourless prisms or tablets, m.p. 109°. Jassoy (Apoth. Zeit., *5*, 150; Abst., 1890, 1154) could not find peucedanin in the roots of *I.Ostruthium*. Merck, however, claims to confirm its presence (Ber.ü.d.Jahr., 1895, 8; Abst., 1897. i, 168).

Schmidt, Jassoy and Haensel (Arch. Pharm., 1898, *236*, 662; Abst., 1899, i, 377) show that "peucedanin" has no definite melting point. They purified it by several extractions with warm ether, when a white gritty residue is left; when the ethereal solution is mixed with a considerable quantity of light petroleum and allowed to stand, "peucedanin" crystallizes in clusters of slender needles. After several repetitions of the process the compound is obtained in slender yellowish needles melting at 99°. It can be obtained perfectly colourless only by repeated crystallization from very dilute solution, when crystals melting sharply at 109° are obtained. They assign the formula $C_{15}H_{14}O_4$ and not $C_{16}H_{16}O_4$, and regard it as the methyl ether of oreoselone. With bromine in chloroform solution it gives monobromo-oreoselone, $C_{14}H_{11}BrO_4$ m.p., 140-141° It gives no acetyl derivative although oreoselone does. The latter gives a phenylhydrazone but the former does not.

Popper (Monatsh., 1898, *19*, 268; Abst., 1898, i, 600) finds that the substances obtained from *Imperatoria Ostruthium* and *P.officinale* are not identical. He finds that imperatorin and peucedanin do not give identical decomposition products, *e.g.*, imperatorin gives on treatment with caustic alkalis oroselone and angelic acid but peucedanin does not give angelic acid. Popper further finds that the substance prepared from *P.officinale*, after crystallization from alcohol and ligroin, is not homogeneous but can be separated into two constituents, differing in their solubility in dry ether. The less soluble portion is $C_{14}H_{11}O_3 . OCH_3$. oroselone-methyl ether, m.p., 105°, b.p., (17 m.m.) 276-281°, which gives oroselone with hydriodic acid. The more soluble part after fractional crystallization from benzene and ether gives yellowish white prisms, m.p., 85-93°. It is probably a mixture of mono-and dimethyl ethers of oroselone.

Herzog and Krohn (Arch. Pharm., 1909, *247*, 553; Abst., 1910, i, 124) have made a comparative examination of the crystalline constituents of the rhizomes of Imperatoria and Peucedanum. Earlier workers have shown that the latter contains peucedanin and oxypeucedanin while the former contains ostruthin and oxypeucedanin, but not peucedanin. The authors extracted Imperatoria with boiling benzene, concentrated the extract and treated with ligroin, obtaining a viscous mass which soon crystallised. The mass is treated with ether, and the oxypeucedanin thus obtained is crystallised successively from acetone, alcohol and chloroform, m.p., 142°. After 14 days the mother liquor gave a new substance ostruthol, m.p., 134.5°, which depresses the melting point of oxypeucedanin. The benzene-ligroin solution contains another new substance osthol, m.p., 84° and ostruthin. Percentage yields are:— oxypeucedanin 1.3, ostruthol 0.3, osthol 0.1 and ostruthin 0.5. Peucedanium extracted by the benzene process gives 2% of peucedanin and 0.3% oxypeucedanin, whilst the roots give 2.5 and 0.5% respectively of the two substances. The oxypeucedanin from Imperatoria is shown to be identical with that from Peucedanum by the mixed melting point method. Oxypeucedanin, $C_{13}H_{12}O_4$, m.p., 142.5°, is optically inactive. HCl gas passed into a concentrated alcoholic solution at 0° and addition of water produces $C_{36}H_{34}O_{11}ClI_2$, m.p., 155.5-157°, the nature of which is unknown. The formula $C_{18}H_{20}O_3$ for ostruthin is confirmed. Osthol, $C_{15}H_{16}O_3$, m.p., 84°, contains one methoxy group. Ostruthol, probably a lactone, is $(C_8H_8O)_8$.

The gum resin known as "galbanum" is the air-dried, milky juice that exudes simultaneously from the trunk and the larger branches of *Peucedanum rubricaule*, Baillon ; *P.galbanifolium* and possibly *P. Schair*, Borszozow, all of which grow principally in Persia. The aromatic, not unpleasant smell of galbanum is due to the large amount of volatile oil which it contains ; yield 10-22% according to the age of the drug. The oil is yellowish, has a specific gravity 0.905-0.955, $\alpha_D + 20°$ to $- 10°$. It contains a dextrogyrate hydrocarbon, $C_{10}H_{16}$, b.p., 160-161°, giving terpin hydrate with nitric acid. Hence it is d-pinene. (See Gildemeister. & Hoffmann, iii, 370). According to Wallach, the fraction 270-280° contains cadinene, $C_{15}H_{24}$, identified by the hydrochloride (Ann., 1887, *238*, 81).

Pimpinella anisum, L., Eng. *Anise or Sweet fennel.* (The Indian names are the same as those for *dill.*)

The plant came originally from the Orient but is now cultivated in almost all parts of the world. Most of the anise distilled comes from Russia. The medicinal properties are the same as those of dill.

The anise fruits owe their smell and taste to their volatile oil, which varies in amount from 1.5 to 3 per cent. This variation is often due to impurities. The residue after distillation of the oil contains 17-19% of protein and 16-22% fat and is therefore prized as a high grade cattle food.

Above 20° the oil is colourless and is congealed by cold to a snow-white crystalline mass. Its properties are:— Sp. gravity (20°) 0.980-0.990, α_D up to $-1°50'$, $n_D^{20°}$ 1.557-1559. It consists principally of two substances, $C_{10}H_{12}O$:— anethol, 80-90% and methyl chavicol. No fenchene is present. Bouchardat and Tardy found p-methoxyphenylacetone (Gildemeister & Hoffmann, iii, 341).

Pimpinellin is the bitter principle of the root of *P.saxifraga* (see Heut Arch. Pharm., 1898, 236, 162. Abst., 1898, i, 598). It crystallizes from dilute alcohol in colourless needles, m.p., 106°, probable formula $C_{14}H_{12}O_5$. Heut also isolated from an alcoholic extract of the plant a yellow crystalline substance, melting at 148°.

Herzog and Hancu simplified the preparation of pimpinellin (Arch. Pharm., 1908, 246, 402; Abst., 1908, i, 905). He arrived at the following conclusions :— Formula $C_{13}H_{10}O_5$, m.p., 119°, probably a lactone, contains two methoxy groups and is oxidised by hydrogen peroxide to a tribasic acid $C_9H_6O_8$, m.p., 220° (decomp.). This acid contains no methoxyl groups and its pyridine salt melts at 179° (decomp.). The second product obtained by Heut is possibly according to these authors, a decomposition product of pimpinellin ; they were, however, unable to isolate it. Vestlin (Abst., 1920, i, 411) obtained in 1.1% yield, a saponin $C_{23}H_{36}O_{18} \cdot 2H_2O$ from the roots of *P.saxifraga.*

Cuminum Cyminum, L., Eng. *Cumin Seed,* Sinh. *Duru or Sudu-duru;* Sans. *Jeeraka, Hrasvangu, Jira, Kunchika, Ajmoda;* Tam. *Shiragam.*

This is principally produced as a commercial article in Morocco, Malta, Syria, the East Indies, Northern India, the Punjab and Persia..

The seeds are used as a medicine and as a spice, Medicinally they are useful in hoarseness, dyspepsia. and chronic diarrhoea. They are regarded as carminative and stomachic and are employed in combination with other drugs for the preparation of many compound medicines for various diseases. Mixed with lime juice, they are useful in cases of bilious nausea in pregnant females. Taken internally shortly after child birth they increase the secretion of milk.

The essential oil distilled from the seeds is known as Oil of Cumin. When fresh it is colourless but later it becomes yellow and even brown. It has the unpleasant bed-bug-like characteristic cumin odour and a spicy somewhat bitter taste. Its physical properties vary with the source of the seeds. Its chief constituent is cuminic aldehyde or cuminal (wrongly called cuminol), cymene and other terpenes. (see Gildemeister & Hoffmann, Volatile Oils iii, 314).

Coriandrum sativum, L., Eng. *Coriander*, Sinh. *Kotthamalli;* Sans. *Kustimbari, Dhanyaka;* Tam. *Kottamalli.*

A herbaceous plant extensively cultivated in all parts of India.

Its fruits are used not only in medicine but also generally as a condiment. It is aromatic, stimulant, carminative, stomachic, antibilious, refrigerant, tonic, diuretic and aphrodisiac. Mohamedan writers describe them as sedative, pectoral and carminative and they prepare an eyewash from it, which is supposed to prevent small-pox from destroying the sight and to be useful in chronic conjunctivitis.

In Ceylon, it is easily the commonest domestic medicine. Decoctions of it either alone or with ginger and *Piper longum* are often given for three days in cases of colds, fevers, influenza, etc. Together with the root of *Aegle marmelos*, it gives a decoction which is given to allay thirst in cases of dysentery, and with *Weniwel* to prevent tetanus.

Coriander was used as a kitchen spice even before the Christian era. Coriander Oil is distilled from the fresh fruit and the exhausted and dried fruits are used as fodder for cattle. They contain 11-17% protein and 11-20% fat. The yield of oil from European fruit varies from 0.8 to 1.0%; the East Indian fruit yields only 0.15-0.2%. The oil is a colourless and faintly yellowish liquid with a characterisitc odour and an aromatic but mild taste and has the following values :—Sp.gr. at 15° 0.870-0.885,

$\alpha_D + 8°$ to $+ 13°$, $n_D^{20°}$ 1.463-1.476. The principal constituent of the oil was recognized by Kawalier (Ann., 1852, *84*, 351) to be a substance of the formula $C_{10}H_{18}O$. Its properties are the same as those of linalool except that it is dextro-rotatory. It is, therefore, the dextro-modification of linalool. It is present to the extent of 70%. There are about 20% of hydrocarbons which comprise the following :—i- α -Pinene, β-pinene, cymene, a very small amount of dipentene, α -and y-terpinenes. In the fractions boiling higher than coriandrol the following were found : higher members of fatty aldehydes, principally n-decylic aldehyde, the alcohols geraniol and borneol and their acetic esters. Oil of Coriander is frequently adulterated with orange oil or turpentine oil. The presence of these oils can be detected by the specific gravity, angle of rotation and insolubility in 70% ethyl alcohol.

Foeniculum vulgare, Gaertn., Sinh. *Maduru or Maha-duru*; Sans. *Madhrika;* Tam. *Sombu,* is a stately plant, native of Europe but now cultivated throughout the East. It is used as a spice and its medicinal properties are the same as those of cumin and caraway. For details see Gildemeister & Hoffmann, ii, 378 and iii 350.

Asafoetida is the inspissated milky juice of several species of *Ferula,* none of which grows in Ceylon. It is called *Perunkayam* in Sinhalese and Tamil and *Hingu* in Sanskrit. It is used by Sinhalese Ayurvedic physicians in dyspepsia, flatulence, colic and diseases of the nervous system. It is also an ingredient in several medicinal oils.

RUBIACEAE

Anthocephalus Cadamba, Miq., Eng. *Wild cinchona;* Sinh. *Ambul-bakmi;* Sans. *Kadamba Nipa, Halipriya (dear to agriculturists), Sisupala (protecting children);* Tam. *Vellai-kadampa.*

A large tree with erect and horizontal branches, found in the low country of Ceylon up to 2000 feet, and also in India, Burma, Sumatra and Borneo. The fruit which is about the size of a small orange is edible.

The juice of the fruit, mixed with cumin and sugar, is given to children in gastric irritability; the fruit is also given in fevers with great thirst. The fresh juice of the bark is applied to the heads of infants when the fontenella sinks, a small quantity mixed with cumin and sugar being also given internally. The bark is also tonic and febrifuge.

Methyl salicylate has been found in the plant. Dymock and others were unable to isolate an alkaloid from the bark.

Adina cordifolia, Hook.f., Sinh. *Kolon;* Tam. *Manchals kadampa,* has the same properties and uses as *Anthocephalu-Cadamba.*

Gardenia latifolia Hit., var luuda, vel arborica, vel gummifera, Sinh. *Galis;* Sans. *Nadi-hingu, Hingu-nadi etc.,* Tam. *Kumbai.*

A small many-stemmed tree or large shrub, growing, in the moist low country of Ceylon ; it is rare. It is also found in Western and Southern India.

The gum which exudes from the fruit is used in medicine and in action is anti-periodic, anthelmintic, alterative and anti-spasmodic. Externally it is antiseptic and stimulant. It is given internally in fevers, dyspepsia, flatulence and chronic skin diseases. The use of the drug by Sinhalese physicians is of recent date. In veterinary practice it is much used to keep off flies from sores and some European physicians have used it is to expel round worms with success.

Gardenia oil is obtained from flowering gardenias by the maceration process from a number of species of *Gardenia.* The whole genus is, however, rare in Ceylon.

Stenhouse and Groves (J. Chem. Soc., 1879, 35, 688) have investigated *G.lucida* from India. They obtained about 100 cc. of essential oil from a hundredweight of resin. Although the resin possessed an alliaceous odour, neither the volatile oil nor the residue did. From the residue they obtained gardenin, $C_{14} H_{12} O_6$ (?) which is oxidized by nitric acid to a red crystalline substance, gardenic acid. Acetyl-and hydro-gardenic acids were prepared but no definite conclusion was reached regarding constitution. The essential oil was fractionated but the fractions were not identified.

Hedyotis auricularia, L., Sinh. *Gete-kola,* is used in deafness. The leaves are applied as an emollient application to abscesses and as a salve for wounds.

Hedyotis fruticosa, L., Sinh. *Weraniya,* is not mentioned in the Nigandus but is used sometimes by Sinhalese physicians.

P.R. Bandarkar (1929 & 1930) has prepared and tested pharmacologically "Hedaurin," which is an extract of *H.auricularia.* In a preliminary report to the South Indian Medical Union of Madras, he states that "this plant known to some families of South Canara as a therapeutic agent, is used as a household remedy, green roots and leaves being boiled in conjee and soup intended for invalids having bowel complaint; also as a general prophylactic, being served periodically in either form to the whole family during the South West Monsoon (June to September), when diarrhoea, dysentery and enteric fever prevail on the west coast. It is also used by some practitioners of indigenous medicine as a decoction of fresh plants in which they dissolve their pills or powders for diarrhoea and dysentery." The preparation (Hedaurin) has been found by him to be useful in colitis and amoebiasis. He further reports that B. B. Dey of Madras has isolated an alkaloid and its hydrochloride in the pure state from the "total alkaloids", and also a possible glucoside.

Ixora coccinea, L., Sinh. *Ratambala,- Ratmal;* Sans. *Raktata, Pathalee, Bandhuka;* Tam. *Vedchi.*

A shrub with long branches and brilliant scarlet flowers, the latter being occasionally yellow. It is one of the commonest and most conspicuous shrubs in Ceylon. The Hindus regard it as sacred to Shiva or Ishwara. (Ixora is a corruption of the latter name.)

The flowers are used as a remedy for dysentery; they are fried in melted butter, rubbed down with a little cumin and *nagakesara* and made into a bolus with sugar candy. The root is also used in dysentery and is a good stomachic and tonic, useful in debility of the stomach.

Ixora parviflora, Vahl., Eng. *Torch tree,* Sinh. *Maharatambala;* Sans. *Iswara;* Tam. *Karankutti.*

A small much-branched tree, common in the dry region of the low country of Ceylon and also in India and Burma. The flowers are pink and sweet-scented. *Ixora zeylanica* is a variety of this.

A decoction of the bark is given in anaemia and general debility. The flowers pounded in milk are given in whooping cough.

Morinda citrifolia, L., and Morinda tinctoria, Roxb., Sinh. *Duhu;* Sans. *Achchhuka;* Tam. *Nuna or Manchavanna.*

These are small trees found in Ceylon, India and Malaya. The former which is a Malayan and Pacific plant is rather rare in Ceylon but is often cultivated. The latter is, however, rather common in the dry region.

It is used medicinally in conjunction with other drugs for fever, dysentery and diarrhoea, and as a tonic. The juice applied externally relieves gout and rheumatism. The root is used as a cathartic. The fruit and leaves in decoction are administered as deobstruent and emmenagogue, also as tonic and febrifuge. The charred leaves are made into a decoction with a little mustard and given in infantile diarrhoea; with aromatics it is used in dysentery. The charred unripe berries, mixed with salt are applied successfully to spongy gums.

Morinda umbellata, L., Sinh. *Kiriwel, Maha Kiriwel*; Tam. *Nuna*, is a scrambling shrub, common in the moist region extending up to 4000 feet or higher throughout Tropical Asia.

The leaves in conjunction with certain aromatics are used in decoction in cases of diarrhoea and dysentery.

The essential oil of *M.citrifolia* has been found to contain as much as 90% of acid (Schimmel's Report, 1909, 78). The essential oil obtained from the fruits of this plant from Java was investigated by Romburgh in 1909 (Abst., 1909, i, 597). Its specific gravity at 13° was 0.927 and was turbid on account of the separation of small crystals, which on crystallization from alcohol melted at 60° and consisted of paraffins. The oil freed from the crystals dissolved almost completely in dilute sodium hydroxide solution. The solution contained caproic and caprylic acids and traces of a higher fatty acid.

The root of *M.citrifolia,* which contains a dye, was first investigated by Thorpe and Smith (J. Chem. Soc. 1888, *53*, 174), who extracted it repeatedly with hot 50% alcohol. The solution was concentrated to half its volume by distillation, filtered, and the filtrate hydrolysed. A precipitate of morindin and morindone, mixed with a large quantity of resin was obtained. The object of the research was, however, to find the nature of morindone.

Perkin and Hummel (J. Chem. Soc., 1893, 63, 1184) examined the root for yellow substances and obtained chlororubin, morindone and traces of yellow substances. They also examined *M.umbellata* (J. Chem. Soc., 1894, *65*, 851). They found that in the general character of the constituents, the root of this plant more closely resembles *madder* than *chay* root, although like the latter it contains only a single colouring matter. Numerous yellow, crystalline substances, totally distinct from those found in chay root, are also present. They isolated morindin, the glucoside of morindone, which was identical with that obtained by Thorpe and others; substances having the following formulae, $C_{16}H_{12}O_6$ possibly a derivative of dimethylanthracene, $C_{16}H_{10}O_5$, possibly hydroxy-methylanthraquinone carboxylic acid; $C_{16}H_{12}O_5$ a monomethyl ether of a trihydroxymethyl anthraquinone; $C_{15}H_{10}O_4$, a dihydroxy-methylanthraquinone; $C_{16}H_{10}O_5$, a hydroxy-methylanthraquinone carboxylic acid and $C_{18}H_{28}O$, in very small quantites.

Oesterle (Arch. Pharm., 1907, *245*, 287; Abst., 1907, ii, 644) obtained by extraction with chloroform the residue from an alcoholic extract of the root of *M.citrifolia* and extracting the residue from the chloroform extract, a substance of the formula $C_{16}H_{12}O_5$, m.p., 216° and having the reactions of a trihydroxy-methylanthraquinone monomethyl ether, possibly identical with emodin monomethyl ether obtained by Perkin and Hummel from the bark of *Ventilago madraspatana.*

A chemical examination of the root and leaves of *M.longiflora* has been carried out by Barrowcliff and Tutin (J. Chem. Soc., 1907, *91*, 1907). No alkaloids were found nor were morindone and morindine detected. A quantity of hydroxy methoxy-methylanthraquinone was isolated and also a small amount of a monomethyl ether of alizarin. Other substances found were resins, formic, acetic, butyric, palmitic and citric acids, a little phytosterol, $C_{27}H_{46}O$, m.p., 130° and a considerable amount of a sugar which yielded d-phenylglucosazone.

Oesterle and Tisza (Arch. Pharm., 1908, *246*, 150; Abst., 1908, ii, 527) confirm the presence of morindin in *M.citrifolia* and records the existence of two substances which were previously found by Perkin and Hummel in *M.umbellata.* The constituents isolated are :—a dihydroxymethylanthraquinone, named soranjidiol, $C_{15}H_{10}O_4$,, m. p., 276°, yielding a diacetyl derivative; an amorphous resin; a substance $C_{16}H_{10}O_5$ identical with

Perkin and Hummel's substance from *M.umbellāta;* an indefinite product morindanigrin resembling those obtained from senna ; a wax $C_{18}H_{28}O$ and a monomethyl ether of a trihydroxy-anthraquinone.

Simonsen, in a Note on the Constituents of *Morinda citrifolia* (J. Chem Soc., 1920, *117*, 561) draws attention to an error in the work of Barrowcliff and Tutin ; the hydroxy methoxy-methylanthraquinone melting at 290° isolated by them is not, as they state, derived from 1.3.dihydroxy-2-methylanthraquinone but is the monomethyl ether of rubiadin. The identity of the constituents of the root bark of two plants as closely related as *M.citrifolia* and *M.longifolia* is of considerable interest. It is possible that the latter at some period of its growth contains morindine, since the quantity of this glucoside appears to vary with the age of the bark. Simonsen examined a specimen of *M.umbellata* which was quite free from colouring matter.

Mussaenda frondosa, L., Sinh. *Mussenda, Wel-buthsarana ;* Sans. *Nagavalli, Srivati ;* Tam. *Vellaelay.*

A scrambling shrub, very common in the moist region up to 4000 feet in Ceylon, India, Andamans and Malaya.

In action it is alterative and demulcent. About 80 grains of the powdered fruit, administered in cow's urine, is said to be a good remedy for jaundice and also for leucoderma. The flowers are used in cough, asthma, ague and flatulence ; externally applied they clean foul ulcers and cure skin eruptions.

Methyl salicylate has been found in the plant. The Pharmacoepia Indica states that all parts of the plant contain a bitter principle having the peculiarities of a glucoside. The aqueous solution of the ether extract of the various parts of the plant contained a yellow colouring matter related to the quercetin group and a colouring matter of the nature of an organic acid was present in the alcoholic extracts, precipitated by acids and redissolving in alkalis giving an orange coloured solution. The fruits gave no alkaloid.

Oldenlandia corymbosa, Linn., Burmanniana, Br. Thw., is an annual and a common weed throughout the Tropics.

O.biflora, L., is rather common, chiefly near the coast.

O.herbacea, Roxb., is very common in dry sandy places up to 4000 feet. These three plants are used by Sinhalese physicians as *Pepiliya,* Sans. *Parpata,* Tam. *Parpadagam.* This is the drug *par excellence* for continued fevers. It is cooling and is especially useful in fever with gastric irritability and in nervous depression. After using it in his practice, Attygalle has found it to be an excellent drug. The authors of the Pharmacographia Indica think that the cooling action is due to the inorganic salts present.

Oldenlandia umbellata, Linn., Eng. *Chaya root,* Sinh. *Saya;* Sans. *Rajana;* Tam. *Saya.*

An annual, common on sandy ground, especially near the coast and in the dry region, and also in South India and North Burma. Its root was at one time an important dyeing material and a Government monopoly.

The leaves are considered expectorant and are used in asthma and phthsis. A 1 in 20 decoction of the root and the leaves is used as a wash for bites of venomous animals. It has also the properties of the three species above.

Perkin and Hummel investigated the colouring and other principles contained in *chaya* root (J. Chem Soc., 1893, 63, 1160 and 1895, 67, 817). In many respects *chaya* root resembles *madder* as both contain ruberythric acid, rubichloric acid and cane sugar, but there are very marked differences in the other constituents of the two roots. Twelve distinct products were isolated by treating the root with sulphurous acid, lime water, alcohol and other solvents. Among them, in addition to those already mentioned, were two dimethyl ethers of anthragallol, alizarin methyl ether and metahydroxy-anthraquinone. It is probable that those substances extracted by sulphurous acid are present in the form of glucoside. On the other hand, those soluble in lime water, *viz.*, m-hydroxy-anthraquinone and hystazarin monomethyl ether are present in the free state only.

Ophiorrhza Mungos, Linn., Eng. *the Mungoose plant* ; Sinh. *Akberiya* ; Sans. *Nagasugandha, Sarpakshi, Patalabhedi* ; Tam. *Keerippundu.*

A common herb growing in sandy places in the moist region from sea-level up to 6000 feet, in Ceylon, India, Burma and Malaya.

The root has a great reputation as a cure for snake bites. Experiments have, however, proved this to be untrue It is merely a bitter tonic.

Paederia foetida, Linn., vel Convulvulus foetidus, Sinh. *Apasumadu* ; Sans. *Prasarani, Apehivata, Gandha-bhadaliya.*

It is found in Central and Eastern Himalayas, Bengal and the Western Peninsula. Although it does not grow in Ceylon, it is used by local physicians as a remedy for rheumatism for which it is regarded almost as a specific.

On steam distillation it gives an essential oil with a highly offensive odour. Dymock and others believe that there are at least two alkaloids, one soluble in and crystallizing from ether and the other slightly soluble in amyl alcohol, chloroform and benzene.

Pavetta indica, Linn., Sinh. *Pavatta* ; Sans. *Siryakphala, Papata, Pappana;* Tam. *Pavaddai.*

It is a bush or small tree, with numerous spreading branches, common in the low country of Ceylon and in India, Burma, Malaya, S. China and N. Australia. It is very variable in its foliage. This is the true *Pavatta* and must not be confounded with *Adathoda* which is also called *Pavatta* in Sinhalese.

It is a bitter tonic and aperient. The root is purgative. It is also regarded as a specific for jaundice. In combination with other drugs it is given in dropsy due to visceral obstructions. The root together with dried ginger is rubbed and given in conjee water in cases of ascites, renal dropsy, etc. Local fomentation with its leaves relieves pain in haemorrhoids. In Malay medicine a decoction of the root is given at child-birth. The leaves in decoction are used as a drink and as a lotion in ulceration of the nose.

Alcohol dissolves the bitter principle of the root. The substance is a glucoside closely related to salicin. (Pharm.Ind.)

Randia Dumetorum, Lam. Eng. *Emetic nut,* Sinh. *Kukuruman ;* Sans. *Madana ;* Tam. *Maruk-kalan-kai.*

A shrub or small tree, very common in the dry region, especially in sandy places near the coast of Ceylon and in Peninsular India, Burma, Java, S. China and Tropical Africa.

The fruit, both rind and pulp, have useful emetic, diaphoretic and antispasmodic properties. It is regarded as the best and safest of emetics, one ripe fruit being sufficient for a dose, expelling phlegm and bile and at the same time acting as an aperient. According to the author of the Supplement to the Indian Pharmacoepia, only the dry pulp and the mucous possess emetic and nauseating properties. It also acts as an astringent and is useful in diarrhoea and dysentery, and the powdered pulp is a good substitute for *Ipececuanha* in dysentery. An infusion of the bark of the root is administered in bowel complaints. The nut, bruised and thrown into pools where there are fish intoxicates them. In colic, the fruit is rubbed to a paste with rice water and applied over the navel.

Randia uliginosa, DC., Sinh. *Et-kukuruman, Wadiga ;* Sans. *Pindaluka ;* Tam. *Wagata.*

A much-branched small tree which is met with in moist places in India and Burma. It is rather rare in Ceylon and is found on the margins of tanks, etc.

The flesh of the large yellow fruit is used in curries, but it is astringent. The unripe fruit is also astringent and is used, roasted in hot ashes after removal of seeds, in diarrhoea and dysentery. The root is sometimes used in similar cases. The plant is described as cooling, sweet and diuretic.

Randia dumetorum has been investigated by Vogtheer (Arch. Pharm., 1894, 232, 489; Abst., 1895, i, 189). He obtained a minute quantity of an alkaloid, which he was unable to characterize or identify. The following substances were also found :—(1) Randiasaponin, a glucoside which forms yellowish plates or a white amorphous powder, m.p., 250° (decomp.). On prolonged hydrolysis with dilute hydrochloric acid it gives randiasapogenin and two sugars, (2) Randic acid, $C_{30}H_{52}O_{10}$, apparently a monobasic acid, crystallizing from alcohol in white nodular masses, m.p., 208-210°. (3) Randiatannic acid, present in small quantities in the pericarp, (4) Randia fat, a yellowish-green butter-like substance, sp. gr. (at 20°,) 0.9175, and saponfication value 160.2 and iodine value (after 2 hours) 43.24.

Rubia cordifolia, Linn., Eng. *Heart-leaved Madder* and *Rubia tinctorum, Linn.*, Eng. *Madder*, Sinh. *Wel-madata, Mandamadiniwel* ; Sans. *Manjistha* ; Tam. *Shevelli, Manjitta.*

These are herbaceous perennial climbers, very common in Ceylon (mountain zone, 3000-7000 feet), India, Java, N. E. Asia and Tropical Africa.

R.cordifolia was formerly considered emmenagogue and diuretic and was used in dropsy, paralysis, jaundice, amenorrhoea and visceral obstructions. It is prescribed by Muslim physicians for paralytic affections, jaundice, obstructions in the urinary passages and amenorrhoea. The fruit is said to be useful in hepatic obstructions. The root in the form of a paste with honey is an application for discolouring, etc. of the skin. It is used as a colouring agent for medicated oils.

Perkin and Hummel (J. Chem. Soc., 1893, 64, 1157) have investigated the allied Indian plant *R.sikkimensis*, which grows in Sikkim and eastward to the Khasia and

Naga Hills. (It was for a long time mistaken for *R.cordifolia.*) The colouring matter of the root of this species cannot be extracted with boiling alcohol as is the case with *R.cordifolia*, and boiling 1% alum solution was used for the purpose. The substances found were purpurin, munjistin, (which was shown to be identical with purpuroxanthin carboxylic acid), a substance, $C_{15}H_8O_6$, (the constitution of which was not determined for want of material) and purpuroxanthin.

" The medical action, if any, is probably due to the small quantity of acrid and resinous matter contained in it ". (Pharm Ind.)

Sarcocephalus cordatus, Miq., Sinh. *Bakmi* ; Tam. *Vammi.*

It is a rather common tree in both the moist and dry regions of the low country of Ceylon. It is found in Malaya and the Philippines but not in Peninsular India. The head of the fruit is succulent and is eaten. It is therefore also called *Kana-bakmi.*

It is not mentioned in the Nigandus but is occasionally used by Sinhalese practitioners.

Spermacoce hispida, L., Eng. " *Shaggy Button Weed* ", Sinh. *Heen-getakola* ; Sans. *Madanaghanta.*

This is very common in the low country of Ceylon and is found throughout India, Malaya and South China.

In action it is alterative and tonic. The seeds are cooling and demulcent and are given in diarrhoea and dysentery. The root is alterative and used like *sarsaparilla.* There is a Hindu myth that an oyster will open its shell if touched by the plant. The plant is eaten as a vegetable.

Webera crymbosa, Willd., Sinh. *Tharana* ; Tam. *Karanai,* is very common up to 7000 feet in Ceylon. The fruit smashed up is applied to boils to promote suppuration.

LYTHRACEAE.

Lagerstroemia Flos-reginae, Retz., Sinh. *Murutha ;* Sans. *Hayakarni, Dirgapatra ;* Tam. *Kadalapuva.*

A large tree with spreading branches and pale, rather smooth bark. It is rather common in the moist low country of Ceylon up to 2000 feet, and also in India, Malaya and China . It is magnificient when in full flower. The wood which is very useful, is light brownish red, hard but not heavy.

It is used in combination with other drugs for various diseases. The root is astringent and the seed is said to be narcotic. The bark and leaves are purgative. In Malaya, a decoction of the bark is given for abdominal pains.

Lawsonia alba, Lam., var L.spinosa, Linn., var L.enermis,, Linn., Sinh. *Marithondii ;* Sans. *Rakta-garbha Mendika ;* Eng. *Henna ; (from Arabic Hinna) ;* Tam. *Maritondi, Aivanam.*

It is cultivated as a hedge plant and is common all over India. It is much esteemed by the Muslims on account of a tradition connected with it and their Prophet. It is seldom used by Sinhalese medical men.

In India its leaves are applied as a poultice to the soles of the feet in " burning of the feet ". A dye obtained from the leaves is extensively used for staining hands and finger nails. An ointment made from the leaves is spoken of as having valuable healing properties, and a decoction is used as an astringent gargle. The bark is given in jaundice and enlargement of the spleen, also in calculous affections, and as an alterative in leprosy and obstinate skin diseases ; in decoction, it is applied to burns, etc. An infusion of the flowers is said to be a good application to bruises. An extract prepared from the flowers and leaves is used by physicians in Southern India as a remedy in lepra, half a teaspoonful twice a day being the dose. A pillow stuffed with the flowers has a reputation of acting as a soporific.

Tommasi (Gazzetta, 1920, 50, i, 263; Abst., 1920, i, 626) isolated the colouring matter Lawsone which forms crystals, m.p., 192-195° (decomp.) and gives an orange-yellow aqueous solution, which undergoes change when boiled. It is fixed well by wool and silk and rapidly and tenaciously by the skin. He assigns the formula $C_{10}H_6O_3$ to it. It is distinctly acid and contains no methoxy groups. It gives a monoacetyl derivative, crystallising in needles melting at 128-130°. Zinc and acetic acid reduce it to a leuco-base which is reconverted into the dye by atmospheric oxygen. By treatment with acetic anhydride and zinc dust it is converted into $C_{16}H_{14}O_6$, nacreous, white laminae, m. p., 134°. The conclusion is drawn that lawsone contains one phenolic hydroxyl group and two quinonic oxygen atoms. Further, since in alcoholic solution it gives with nickel acetate an intense red colouration and after some hours a deposit of garnet-red crystals, the substance must be regarded as a hydroxy-naphthaquinone and is probably identical with 2.hydroxy - 1: 4-naphthaquinone.

Punica granatum, Eng. *Pomegranate,* Sinh. *Delum ;* Sans. *Kuchappala, Shukadana ;* Tam. *Madalan-kai.*

A small ornamental tree with large scarlet flowers, natives of Northern Africa and Southern Europe. It is commonly cultivated in gardens throughout the East. The fruit is of the size of a large apple with a tough rind, of a bright red orange colour when ripe and crowned with persistent calyx lobes. The succulent juicy coating of the numerous seeds is of a sweet acid taste, sometimes very tart and astringent. The Tropical fruit is inferior to that of its original home.

This is largely used in medicine. The fruit has long been esteemed as food and medicine. The rind of the fruit is very astringent and is used in combination with other drugs in the treatment of dysentery. The juice of the pulp covering the seeds is considered cooling and is given, mixed with saffron, as a cooling medicine. The root bark is used as an anthelmintic. For haemorrhoids the juice of the green fruit is given rubbed with galls, cloves and ginger in honey.

The root bark was first investigated by Tanret (Compt. rend., 1878, *86*, 1270) who isolated four alkaloids from it. (See also Compt. rend., 1879, *88*, 716; 1880, *90*, 696). Piccinini (Gazzetta, 1899, *29*, ii, 311) isolated a fifth. Two of Tanret's alkaloids, pelletierine and methyl-pelletierine, are optically active, the third iso-pelletierine is inactive. The work of Hess and Eichel (Ber., 1917, *50*, 1386) reduced the number of alkaloids to three :—Pelletierine $C_8H_{15}ON$ (Tanret's isopelletierine), pseudo-pelletierine, $C_9H_{15}ON$ and methyl-isopelletierine $C_9H_{17}ON$ (Tanret's methyl pelletierine and Piccinini's iso-methylpelletierine.) Hess and Eichel later added two more, isopelletierine $C_8H_{15}ON$ and α-N-methyl-piperidyl-2-propan-β-one $C_9H_{17}ON$. The alkaloids were prepared by extracting a finely ground mixture of the bark and slaked lime with chloroform, and the solution thus obtained with hydrochloric acid. The acid extract is made alkaline with caustic soda and extracted with ether and the ethereal solution dried over potash. Pelletierine and methyl-iso-pelletierine distil at 100-120° (15-20mm. press.) and pseudo-pelletierine at 145°. The formula of Pelletierine is

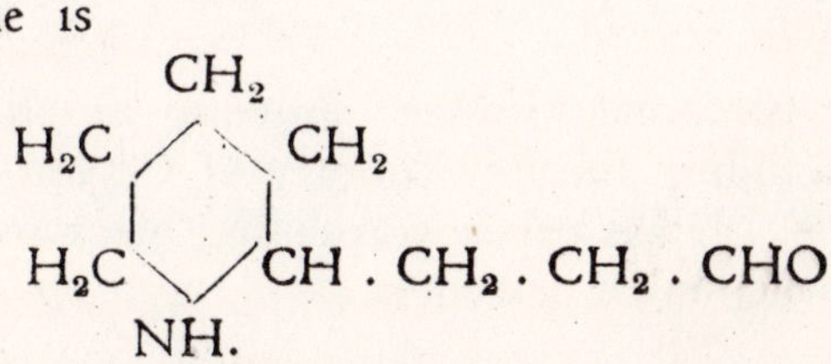

For a fuller account, see Henry's Plant Alkaloids. (pp. 39-48).

Pomegranate root bark is officinal in the U.S.A. Pharmacoepia but is now little used in medicine. The active principle is said to be pelletierine, which is highly toxic to tape-worms, hence the use of the bark as a vermifuge. A crude mixture of pelletierine tannate and sulphate is officinal in the British and U. S. A. Pharmacoepias.

The yellow colouring principles of the Tannin matter of the rind of the pomegranate have been investigated by Perkin (J. Chem. Soc., 1897, *71*, 1137).

Woodfordia floribunda, Sal., Sinh. *Militta* ; Sans. *Dhataki, Dhauri, Agnijvala* ; Tam. *Dhatari-puspam.*

A straggling shrub, rare, and grows in open sunny places in the lower mountain region of Ceylon, and also in India, China, Tropical Africa and Madagascar. It is a native of Mauritius. In Ceylon, it flowers in March and April (bright brick red). The Sinhalese medical men use Myla flowers (*Bauhinia racemosa*) as a substitute.

In action the flowers are stimulant and astringent ; when dry they are astringent and tonic. They are added to Aristas to cause alcoholic fermentation. They are also used in dysentery and other bowel complaints and irritant haemorrhage. The powder is given with honey in leucorrhoea.

The flowers contain 20.6% tannic acid, hence their use as a mordant.

LEGUMINOSEAE

Abrus precatorius, L., Jequirity, Eng. *Indian or Jamaica Liquorice,* Sinh. *Olinda* ; Sans. *Gunja* ; Tam. *Kuntumani.*

A slender perennial climber growing in all Tropical countries, including the low country of Ceylon, especially the dry region. It has pretty scarlet and black seeds, which are used as weights by jewellers.

The leaves are steeped in warm mustard oil and applied over the seat of pain or are warmed over the fire and applied after smearing the part with warm castor oil. The fresh juice of the leaves mixed with some bland oil relieves pain and reduces swellings when applied to the painful part. A paste made of the leaf juice and plumbago root (Sinh. *Ratnitul*) applied for a month is said to remove leucoderma. Chewing the leaves and swallowing the juice relieves hoarseness. The seeds are poisonous but are used internally in nervous affections in combination with other drugs ; when powdered and boiled with milk they have a powerful tonic and aphrodisiac action. If administered uncooked they are strongly purgative and emetic, and in larger doses they produce poison with symptoms similar to cholera. When decorticated and finely ground they are useful for granular eyelids and pannus ; they produce inflammation of the conjuctiva. Sloane, in 1700, appears to have been the first to suggest the use of *abrus* root as a substitute for liquorice.

The seeds contain two poisonous proteins, one a globulin and the other an albumose. Martin (British Med. Journ., 1889, *2*, 184 ; Abst., 1889, *11*. 1026) found that the globulin is soluble in 15% salt solution, coagulates between 75° and 80° and is precipitated by saturating the solution with sodium chloride or magnesium sulphate. The albumose is soluble in water, is not precipitated by boiling and gives the biuret reaction and the characteristic nitric acid reaction of the albumoses. Both these proteins produce nearly the same effects, *viz.*, local oedema and ecchymosis and gastroenteritis. There is a gradual sleepiness ending in coma and rapid onset of rigor mortis. They have a remarkable lowering effect on the body temperature. The globulin produces rapid breathing while the albumose does not have this effect to the same degree. The activity of both proteins is destroyed at a temperature below 100°, the globulin between 75° and 80°, the albumose at 85°. Between 50 and 80° the activity is diminished.

Karl Brown (Chem. Zeitung, 1903, *29*, 32 ; Abst., 1905, ii, 113) found that the aqueous extracts of the seeds lessened the rate of hydrolysis of castor oil.

Sarkar (Biochem. J., 1914, 8, 281 ; Abst., 1914, ii, 1162) has found that the outer layer of the seed coats is impermeable to water and other solvents. On soaking the crushed seed coats in water two colouring matters, yellow and scarlet, are extracted and can be separated by shaking with ether. The scarlet, which predominates, remains dissolved in water and can be purified by means of its insoluble calcium salt. The scarlet colouring matter is located in the outermost layer of the cells.

The Pharmacographia Indica contains a detailed account of experiments on the physiological action of the drug.

Acacia. There are many varieties or species of Acacia, all of which yield a gum resin which is used both medicinally and for various economic purposes.

Acacia arabica, Willd., Eng. *Gum arabic* ; Sinh. *Babboola* ; Sans. *Vabbula* ; Tam. *Karuvel.*

A small tree or shrub of India, Egypt, Tropical Africa and North Ceylon and is one of the sources of gum arabic. The astringent bark is extensively used in India for tanning and also as a dye in calico printing The plant is employed in India for making charcoal for gunpowder.

Acacia catechu, Willd., Eng. *Cutch or Catechu, Khair or Katha of India* ; Sans. *Khadira* ; Sinh. *Kayippu* ; Tam. *Voadalam, Karangalli, Kasku-kutta.*

A medium-sized tree common in parts of India and Burma. A black gum resin is obtained by boiling the chips of the heart wood. It is astringent and extensively used for dyeing and tanning. It is also chewed with betel. Either in the form of a powder or tincture, it is a valuable astringent in passive diarrhoeas and haemorrhages, especially in children. It relieves hoarseness, sore throat, loss of voice, etc. when a small piece is allowed to dissolve slowly in the mouth. The tincture is an excellent application for threatened bed sores.

Acacia sundra, DC., Sinh. *Rat-keeriya* ; Sans. *Khadira* ; *Raktha chandana* ; Tam. *Kodali-murunkai.*

A small or middle-sized tree, with dark brown bark, growing in the dry region of Ceylon, but is rare. It also occurs in Peninsular India and Burma. "This is so closely allied to *A.catechu*, Willd., as to be combined with it by many botanists. That tree, however, has more numerous pinnae and leaflets and the calyx is tomentose" (Trimen).

Greshoff (Ber., 1890, *23*, 3537; Abst., 1891, i, 336) isolated from *Acacia tenerrima* (which is not found in Ceylon) a bitter and poisonous alkaloid easily soluble in chloroform and ether. The lethal dose for bufo is 3 mgm. This is the first alkaloid found in a plant of this genus.

The gum of *A.decurrens* (not found in Ceylon) contains, according to Stone (Am. Chem. J., 1895, *17*, 196; Abst., 1895, ii, 285) a complex carbohydrate of the galacto-araban character and does not differ essentially from gum arabic, peach gum or cherry gum.

Perkin and Yoshitake (J. Chem Soc., 1902, *81*, 1160) have investigated *acacia* and *gambier catechus*, the former from *A.catechu*. They obtained three eatechins from them :— (1) m.p., 204-205° (2) m.p., 175-177° (3) m.p., 235-237°. All give the phloroglucinol reaction. Although their general reactions are the same, they are distinct substances. Perkin (J. Chem. Soc., 1905, *87*, 398) advances further evidence for the opinion expressed in the previous paper that the catechins obtained are isomeric reduction products of quercetin.

Steel (Chem. News, 1921, *123*, 315; Abst. 1922, i, 310) has found 18.8% (on dry weight) of calcium oxalate (hydrated) in the outer and inner bark of *A.cambagei*, whilst the outer white wood contains 5.81% and the inner dark-wood 3.81%. Samples of the bark from other species of *Acacia* contained amounts of oxalate varying from 1.36 to 8.92%.

The essential oils from *A.faranesiana, Willd.*, indigenous to the West Indies and West Africa, *A.Cavenia,* Hook & Arm., cultivated in South France, are described in Gildemeister & Hoffmann, ii, 588-592.

Adenanthera pavonina, Sinh. *Madathiya ;* Sans. *Kuchandana ; Tilaka, Raktaya ;* Tam. *Anaikuntamani.*

A quick-growing tall tree, common in the low country of Ceylon and in India, Malaya, China and the Philippines. The bright scarlet seeds are the principal weights used by goldsmiths ; a seed weighs somewhat less than four grains.

Powdered seeds externally applied hasten suppuration. The bark is used in decoction for fever and other diseases and is also useful in haemorrhage from the bowels and haematuria. Decoction of the leaves is a remedy for chronic rheumatism and gout. It also acts as aphrodisiac.

Albizzia odoratissima, Benth., Sinh. *Sooriya-mara, Huriyi ;* Sans. *Sirisa, Sukapriya ; Suka-pushpa, Suka-druma ;* Tam. *Pannai-murunkai.*

A very large tree, with thick, grey, rough bark and spreading branches, common in the low country of Ceylon and in India and Malacca. Its heart-wood is dark-brown, very hard and works and seasons well.

In medicine it is regarded as tonic and alterative. Powdered bark with melted butter is an excellent tonic and alterative. The seeds are prescribed in spermatorrhoea and malaria.

Bauhinia tomentosa, L., Sinh. *Kaha-petan, Petan ;* Sans. *Phalgu ;* Tam. *Tiruvatti,* is a small tree or large shrub, with slender branches and yellow flowers.

The plant is anti-dysenteric and anthelmintic. The decoction of the root bark is useful in hepatitis. The dried leaves, buds and flowers are prescribed in dysentery.

Butea frondosa, Koen. ex Roxb., Eng. *Bastard oak;* Sinh. *Kela; Gas-kela ;* Sans. *Palasha ;* Tam. *Parasu, Murukkan maram.*

An erect tree with large, leathery, broad trifoliate leaves, indigenous to the forests of the dry region of India, Ceylon and Burma. It bears in the dry months a profusion of beautiful crimson or orange-scarlet flowers. It also furnishes a resin and a useful fibre from the bark. A lac is produced on the young twigs. The tree is held sacred by the Hindus.

The gum, known as "butea" gum or *Bengal Kino*, is used in tanning. Medicinally it is astringent and is well-adapted to children and delicate females ; it is useful in dysentery. The seeds are anthelmintic (which has been confirmed experimentally by Dymock and others) and is also used externally for ringworm. They are also laxative and are given in combination with other drugs to expel worms. Pieces of the bark chewed with sugar candy relieve thirst.

The chemistry of the colouring matter of the flowers of *B.frondosa* has been worked out by Perkin and Hummel (J. Chem Soc., 1904, *85*, 1459). Previously, in 1894, Hummel and Cavallo had isolated a substance, butein, $C_{15}H_{14}O_5$, which they thought was the colouring matter. Hill (1903) extracted a colouring matter in the form of small, lemon-yellow crystals which gave the reactions of fisetin. He also noticed a tannin.

Perkin changed the name butein to butin as the substance is not the colouring matter. Butin crystallises in small colourless needless, m.p., 224-226°, formula $C_{15}H_{12}O_5$. The air-dried product is $C_{15}H_{12}O_5 \cdot \frac{1}{2}H_2O$. It gives a triacetyl derivative, m.p., 123-125° and a tribenzoyl, m.p., 155- 157°. Butin dissolves readily in cold solutions of alkali, forming a pale orange liquid which, when acidified, deposits the unchanged substance. On boiling with potassium hydroxide solution and acidifying, a bright orange crystalline precipitate separates out, which is butein, m.p., 213-215°, from dilute alcohol, formula $C_{15}H_{12}O_5 \cdot H_2O$. It gives a tetra-acetyl derivative, m.p., 129-131°. Both butin and butein give on fusion with potash, resorcinol and protocatechuic acid. The two substances were methylated and methylation products studied and synthesized. The following formulae have been assigned :—

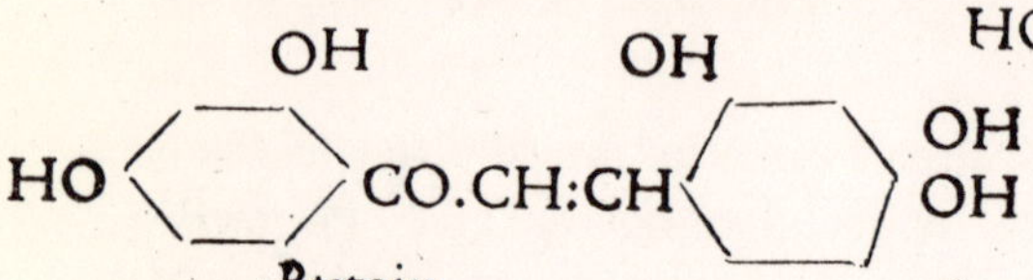

Butein

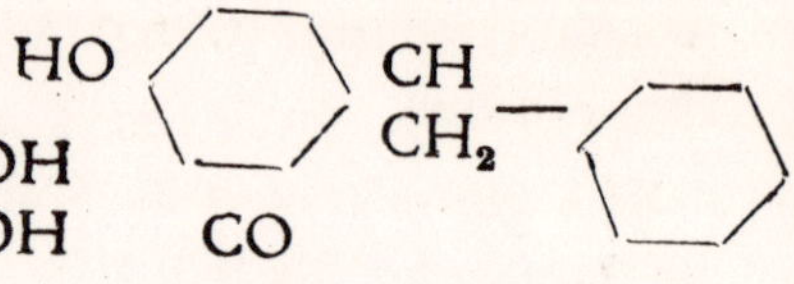

Butin

The oil of the seeds is yellow, nearly tasteless, solidifies at 10° and has sp. gr. 0.917. (Lepine).

Caesalpinia Bonducella, Roxb., Eng. *Nicker tree, Bonduc nut* ; Sinh. *Kumburuwel* ; Sans. *Putikaranja, Latakaranja, Kubberakshi* ; Tam. *Punnaikkalaichi*.

A stout climbing shrub, with very hard globular or ovoid seeds. It is common throughout India and Ceylon.

The seeds have been used in medicine in India for a long time. They are regarded as anthelmintic, bitter-tonic, febrifuge and anti-periodic. The roots and leaves are deobstruent, emmenagogue and febrifuge. Rubbed into a paste the seed is given in colic with long pepper for malarial fever. The seeds roasted and powdered are given internally for hydrocele and are also applied externally, spread over castor leaves. A common domestic remedy for colic and vomitting in children (with a suspicion of worms) is to give the tender leaves of *Bonduc* fried in ghee. The oil expressed from the seeds is used in India as a cosmetic as it is said to soften the skin and remove pimples. (J. Indian Chem. Soc., 1930, 7, 207).

Caesalpinia digyna, Rottl., Sinh. *Wakirimul* ; Hind. *Vakarimul*, is a woody climber very rare in Ceylon, found also in India and Malaya.

The powdered root mixed with milk, ghee, cumin and sugar is given in phthsis and scrofula. The powder is also astringent and given in diarrhoea.

Caesalpina Sappan, L., Eng. *Sappan wood* ; Sinh. *Patangi* Sans. *Patanga, Rukta-mukta* ; Tam. *Parthangi vattangi*.

A very ancient introduction to Ceylon and is a native of India and Malaya ; it is frequently met with in a semi-wild state or planted as a fence. It was formerly much cultivated as a dye-wood for export. The colouring matter, sappan, is red and resembles haemotoxylin.

It is very little used in medicine. Its decoction acts as emmenagogue and is also used in diarrhoea and dysentery. In China, it is supposed to have a special affinity for the blood ; (the belief is undoubtedly based on the Doctrine of Signatures). It is used consequently as a vulnerary for wounds, haemorrhages and disturbance of the menstrual functions. It is also used as astringent and sedative.

Perkin (J. Chem. Soc., 1897, *71*, 1137) has investigated the value of the seed pods of *Caesalpinia coriaria* (not found in Ceylon) as a tanning material.

The colouring matter of sappanwood appears from Bolley's investigations to be identical with Chevreul's brazilin obtained from brazilwood. Pure sappan red or brazilin, $C_{16}H_{14}O_5$, crystallises from absolute alcohol in colourless rhombohedra or monoclinic prisms. It is oxidised to brazilein.

Canavalia ensiformis, DC., Eng. *Sword-Jack or Horse-bean ;* Sinh. *Wal-awara ;* Sans. *Mahashibee ;* Tam. *Koli-awarai.*

A perennial twiner or creeper (there is also a bush form) bearing coarse, rather flat, sword-shaped pods with large seeds. The young pods and seeds are eaten as a vegetable.

The root ground into a paste with cow's urine and administered internally for several days is said to cure enlargement of the liver.

The proteins of this bean have been investigated by several workers. Johns and Jones (J. Biol. Chem., 1916, 24) extracted a globulin of the following percentage composition, C 52.36, H 6.90, N 16.29, S 0.40. Subsequently (ibid., page 67) he separated two globulins by fractional precipitation with ammonium sulphate, *viz.*, canavalin and concanavalin. After removal of the globulins an albumin of the legumelin type was also isolated.

In 1919 Sumner (J. Biol. Chem., 1919, *37*, 137) obtained two crystalline globulins. Wester (Rec. trav. chim., 1921, *40*, 320) obtained from the beans a urease, specific in its action, which did not decompose the disubstituted carbamides examined by them.

Cassia Absus, Sinh. *Boo-thora* ; Tam. *Mulaippalavirai, Kuttikkol, Edikkol, Karunkanam*, is an erect annual, common especially in the dry region of the low country of Ceylon and found throughout the Tropics of the Old World.

Mohammedan writers describe the seeds as attenuant and astringent, and believe that they strengthen the sight when used as a collyrium. In purulent conjunctivitis about a grain of the powdered seeds after being boiled is introduced beneath the eyelids. The seeds are also a useful application on ringworm.

Cassia alata, Linn., Sinh. *Et-tora* ; Sans. *Dadhrugna* ; Tam. *Pannan, Takarai.*

This tree is not a native of India but is an introduction from the West Indies, where it has a reputation as a remedy for ringworm and is used internally to promote expectoration, the action of the bowels and the excretion of urine. The evidence collected by physicians in India points to the efficacy of this drug. The best way of applying it is to bruise the leaves and mix them with lime juice, the paste thus prepared being spread upon the affected part. On account of their purgative action the leaves have been used in the same manner as *senna*. It is largely used in Malayan medicine for similar purposes.

Cassia auriculata, Linn., Sinh. *Ranawara* ; Sans. *Akuli* ; *Saradi* ; Tam. *Avirai.*

It grows in India and Ceylon. Its bark is about as thick as cinnamon and tastes sweet and moderately astringent.

The small, flat, pleasant-tasted heart-shaped seeds of this species are reckoned among refrigerators and attenuants and are prescribed in electuary, in cases in which the habit is preternaturally heated, or depraved. (Ainslie). The powder of the seed, blown into the eye, is valuable in certain stages of opthalmia. The use of the seeds as an application on the eyes in chronic, purulent conjunctivitis is spoken of favourably. The root is used in decoction as an alterative. From the flowers a "tea" is prepared which is prescribed in diabetes. A compound syrup is prepared with the flowers, mocharas, and Indian *Sarsaparilla* and is prescribed for nocturnal emissions. The seeds are also used in diabetes, a compound powder made with all parts of the plant being considered a specific.

Clitoria ternatea, Linn., Sinh. *Katarodu ;* Sans. *Aparajita, Gokarna, Ashpota, Vishnukranti;* Tam. *Karuttappu, Kakkanankodi.*

A common, perennial, twining herb, growing perfectly wild in the dry region of Ceylon and throughout the Tropics. The flowers are intensely bright blue, often much larger in cultivation, and are sometimes white.

The fresh root has an acrid, bitter taste and is described as laxative and diuretic. It is usually given in combination with other drugs ; even by itself it is a safe and good purgative. It is a useful drug in case of snake-bite. The variety with white flowers is used for that purpose and the expressed juice of the fresh flowers is mixed with human milk and a teaspoonful is poured into each nostril ; for bites of rats and mice the variety with blue flowers appears to be used, a decoction of the roots prepared with water or cow's milk given with sugar and continued once a day for several weeks. The juice of the root of the white-flowered variety is blown up the nostrils as a remedy for hemicrania.

Ether extracts a yellow resin soluble in alcohol and alkaline solutions and the residue in extraction with alcohol gives an amorphous, reddish-brown acid resin. This resin forms 4% of the root bark. No alkaloid has been detected. (Pharm. Ind.).

Crotalaria juncea, L., Eng. *Sunn or San Hemp* ; Sinh. *Hàna* ; Sans. *Sana* ; Tam. *Shanal*, is an erect annual, 6-10 feet high, with bright yellow flowers. It is indigenous to Tropical Asia generally ; it occurs commonly in Ceylon in the dry region. It is cultivated for the strong and useful fibre obtained by retting the stems.

The seeds and leaves are used in medicine and are said to be cooling and to purify the blood. It is given in cases of fever and skin diseases. It is, however, less commonly used than *C.verrucosa*.

Crotalaria verrucosa, L., Sinh. *Nilandunkiriya* ; Sans. *Dhavani* ; *Sanapushpi* ; Tam. *Kilvenlappa*.

A large much-branched herb, a common weed in open ground in the low country of Ceylon and throughout the Tropics.

The juice of the tender leaves is used both internally and externally for scabies and impetigo. A poultice of the leaves is applied to discharging eruptions of the skin so as to clean them before applying curative medicines.

Greshof (Ber., 1890, 23, 3537) has found that the leaves of *C.retusa*, (Sinh. *Kahaandunkiriya*, Tam. *Kilukilippi*), contain considerable quantities of indican and that the seeds contain an alkaloid, which is found in larger quantities in the seeds and leaves of *C.striata, L.*, which is also a common Ceylon weed. The base is a strong poison and is probably related to the known alkaloids of other *Genistae*.

Derris uliginosa, Benth., Sinh. *Kalawel*, is a strong woody climber, common in the low country near the sea coast, chiefly in the dry region and also found in India, China and other tropical regions.

The bark is used as a fish poison and also to kill worms and insects which infest leaves and flowers. In medicine it is given as an alterative for rheumatism, paralysis and dysmenorrhoea in the form of a ghrita ; with asafoetida, garlic and plumbago root it used externally in rheumatism.

Derris elliptica, Benth., is largely used in Java in fishing and appears also to be a constituent of the Borneo arrow poison. A 1 in 300,000 decoction of the root in water is fatal to fish. Greshoff (Ber., 1890, 23, 3537) isolated a substance "derrid" which does not contain nitrogen and is not a glucoside. On fusion with potash it gave salicylic and protocatechuic acids. It occurs almost exclusively in the cortex of the root but Greshoff was unable to obtain it pure.

van Sillevoldt (Abst., 1900, i, 109) assigns the formula $C_{33}H_{30}O_{10}$ to derride which he prepared from the root of *D.elliptica*, as a pale yellow substance, m.p., 73°, by treating with water, extracting with alcohol, evaporating the alcoholic solution and treating the residue with ether. On boiling with alcoholic HCl it gives an anhydride $C_{33}H_{28}O_9$, which is also present in crude derride and is not dissolved by ether. It forms small needles melting at 214° and gives with hydriodic acid a substance of the formula $C_{30}H_{19}O_6(OH)_3$, m.p., 240°.

Power (Pharm., 1903, 6, 1; Abst., 1903, ii, 323) investigated the Chemistry of the Stems of *Derris uliginosa*. The bark yields 9.3% tannic acid, equivalent to 6.3 % in the whole stem. The stem also contains gum, sugar, potassium nitrate, hexoic, arachidic and stearic acids, ceryl alcohol, two isomerides of cholesterol and two resins, one soluble and the other insoluble in chloroform. The toxic effect of the plant is due to some constituent (probably) of the resin soluble in chloroform.

Lenz has also examined the constituents of the Derris species. *D.elliptica* from New Guinea does not contain any alkaloid. Derrin is best extracted from the roots by means of boiling benzene. It crystallizes from alcohol in small colourless plates, m.p., 158°. It is toxic to fish. Stuhlmani bark from German East Africa was also examined and found to contain no alkaloid.

Desmodium triflorum, DC., Sinh. *Heen-undupiyali;* Tam. *Sirupullady,* is a very small perennial herb, with numerous long, slender, prostrate branches rooting at the nodes. It is very common in the low country of Ceylon up to 2000 feet or more and throughout the Tropics. It is an abundant and valuable constituent of turf in Ceylon, standing drought very well.

The leaves, well washed and ground with cow's milk are taken daily as galactagogue by women after confinement. They are also administered to children as a remedy for diarrhoea caused by indigestion, and in convulsions. The fresh plant, well bruised, is applied to wounds that do not heal readily.

Desmodium heterophyllum, DC., Sinh. *Maha-undupiyali;* Tam. *Sirupullady,* is a perennial herb having numerous, prostrate, slender stems rooting at lower nodes, densely covered with spreading hairs. It is very common in the low country like the preceding and is also found throughout India and Malaya and in China and the Philippines.

Both these are used in medicine. Their roots are considered carminative, tonic and diuretic and are used in bilious complaints. The leaves of both are galactagogue. The other properties are the same as those of *D.triflorum.*

Desmodium gangeticum, DC., is *Salaparni* of the Sanskrit writers. It is called *Aswenna* by the Sinhalese but there has been some controversy regarding the identity of *Aswenna* with *D. gangeticum.*

D. gangeticum is of interest as being one of the *Dasamula Kvatha* of Ayurvedic medicine. It is placed among the five minor plants of the Dasamula (ten roots). The root is described as alterative and tonic, and a remedy for vomiting, fever, asthma and dysentery.

No alkaloids or other active principles have been isolated although the Pharmacographia Indica records some properties of aqueous, alcoholic and other extracts of the root.

Dichrostachys cinerea, W. & A., Sinh. *Andara, Katu-andara;* Sans. *Sarawirataru, Dirghamula;* Tam. *Vadatara, Vidattal.*

A shrub or small tree with numerous branches, very common, in the dry region and in barren places in Ceylon, India, Malay Islands and Tropical Africa.

It is sometimes given for fever in combination with other drugs and used also in venomous snake bites.

Entada scandens, Benth., Eng. *Gilla nuts;* Sinh. *Puswel;* Sans, *Gilla.*

An immense woody climber, with a thick trunk and twisted snake-like branches. It is common in the low country of Ceylon up to 2000 feet and throughout the Tropics. Certain hill tribes of India use the seeds as a soap to wash their hair.

The juice of the wood and bark is used as an external application to ulcers. A paste of the seeds is applied to relieve inflammatory glandular swellings and in pains of the joints and loins and in swollen hands and feet in cases of general debility. The kernel of the seed ground down to a paste with honey is applied to the eyes for venomous snake bites. It is also said to be an emetic, when given internally. In India, the seeds are used as soap to wash the hair.

The saponins of the seeds have been examined by Rosenthaler (Arch. Pharm., 1903, 241, 614; Abst., 1904, ii, 72). The powdered seeds were freed from fat with ether and then extracted with alcohol. The alcoholic extract was cooled and mixed with ether. The substance that separated was dissolved with barium hydroxide solution. The small precipitate formed was suspended in water, decomposed with carbon dioxide, filtered, and the filtrate evaporated to dryness. A small amount of a saponin, (a), formed a lather with water and was decomposed by boiling with dilute acids giving an insoluble sapogenin and a solution which reduced Fehling's solution. From the barium hydroxide solution another substance, entada saponin, (b), was obtained and purified. It was amorphous and contained ash 1.6/; C 49.7, H 6.1%, corresponding approximately to the formula $C_{15}H_{22}O_{10}$. It forms a triacetyl derivative and is hydrolysed by 10% HCl, yielding galactose and a crystalline sapogenin $C_{30}H_{50}O_6$ and an amorphous substance.

Erythrina indica, Lam., Eng. *Indian coral tree, Moochy wood tree;* Sinh. *Erabadu;* Sans. *Mimbataru, Mandara, Parijataka, Paribhadra;* Tam. *Mullu-murukku.*

A tree attaining to a large size, with thin, smooth, grey bark. It is very common in the low country and much planted. It is also found throughout India, Malaya, Java and Polynesia. The brilliant scarlet flowers are produced when the branches are bare of leaves, hence the name coral tree.

The juice of the leaves is applied to syphilitic buboes and is also given mixed with castor oil for dysentery. With a few drops of honey the fresh juice is a good vermifuge, whether for round, tape or thread worms. It is injected into the ear for relieving earache and is also an anodyne for toothache. The bark is febrifuge and its juice kills maggots in foul ulcers. It is also used as a lactagogue and an emmenagogue. It is an ingredient in many decoctions.

The Pharm. Ind. gives the following account: " The first physiological experiments made with the bark of this tree were those of Bochefontaine and Rey, who communicated the results arrived at by them to the Academie des Sciences in 1881; they concluded that the drug acts upon the central nervous system so as to diminish or abolish its functions. Pinet and Duprat resumed the study of the action of this drug upon frogs in 1886, and communicated the following results to the Societe de Biologie :— One centigram of the watery extract of the bark was introduced under the skin of the right leg of a frog weighing 30 grams. This caused considerable local irritation, but at the end of 25 to 30 minutes the frog remained motionless; placed on its back it remained in that position, only occasionally making slight spontaneous movements: if a limb were pinched only very feeble reflex movements were induced. When the left sciatic nerve was excited by a Pulvermacher's clamp, the distant end of the divided nerve responded to the stimulus, whilst the near end was hardly affected. The electric contractability of the muscles was diminished, and reflex action abolished. Respiration became very slow and was sometimes suspended. Moreover, the heart was observed to dilate very slowly, and the ventricle at the time of the systole, which had become imperfect, assumed a folded appearance, and at the diastole the heart presented a marbled appearance, pale in some places and red in others. The strength of the contractions was not much affected."

Greshoff (Ber., 1890, 23, 3540) has investigated the chemistry of *Erythrina* (Stenotropis) *Broteroi Hassk*, from the Dutch East Indies. The cortex of the plant has a large quantity of alkaloid, which was prepared by Stas' method and was found to be soluble in ether. Its sulphate crystallizes from aqueous solutions. It gives precipitates with mercuric chloride, gold chloride, platinum chloride, potassium thiocyanate, potassium dichromate, picric acid, iodine solution, tannin, etc. It is somewhat strongly poisonous. It is also recorded that the seeds of *Erythrina* (Hypaphorus) *subumbrans Hassk.*, contain a poisonous alkaloid most easily isolated as a metallic double salt.

Weehuizen (Abst., 1907, ii, 905) has detected nitrous acid in the leaves of *Erythrina* which had been macerated and put aside for a short time. Nitrous acid was not found when the enzyme was killed by immersion of the leaves in boiling water. It is inferred that the acid is liberated from a glucoside by the action of an enzyme.

Betting (Abst., 1909, ii, 924) crushed 100 grams of the leaves of a variety of *Erythrina,* gently heated it in a generating flask on a water bath, drew purified air through it by means of an aspirator and obtained 0.03% of nitrous anhydride. Acetone was also given off.

Cohen (Abst., 1909, ii, 925) found formic, oleic linoleic, palmitic and behenolic acids in the fat obtained from the seeds of *Erthrynia hypaphorus subumbrans.* The unsaponifiable part contained sitosterol and two other cholesterols, either identical with or closely related to stigmasterol and brassicasterol.

Glycyrrhiza glabra, Linn. Eng. *Liquorice ;* Sinh. *Welmee;* Sans. *Yashtimadhu, Madhuka;* Tam. *Ati-maduram.*

This tree grows in Arabia, Persia, Afghanistan and Turkey it is cultivated in the Punjab, Sindh and Peshawar. The root is imported into Ceylon .

The root has been used in medicine from a remote period and is prescribed in inflammatory affections, thirst and hoarseness. It is an ingredient in decoctions for fever, dysentery and many other ailments.

According to Fluckiger and Hanbury, liquorice root, contains in addition to sugar and albuminous matter, a peculiar sweet substance named glycyrrhizin, which is precipitated from a strong decoction by the addition of acid, or cream of tartar solution, or neutral or basic lead acetate. It is an amorphous powder having a strong bitter-sweet taste and an acid reaction. Its solution in hot water gelatinizes on cooling. Gorup-Besanez (1861) suggests $C_{24}H_{36}O_9$ as the most probable formula. On hydrolysis with dilute hydrochloric acid it gives a resinous amorphous bitter substance, glycyrettin, and an uncrystallisable sugar, probably glucose.

Haensel (Abst., 1900, i, 107) obtained liquorice oil in 0.03% yield by distilling Spanish liquorice root. The Russian root gave 0.035%. These oils have a feeble acid reaction, possibly due to glycyrrhizic acid, but their composition is not identical, the Russian oil being dextro, and the Spanish oil laevo-rotatory.

Mimosa pudica, Linn. Eng. *Sensitive plant;* Sinh. *Nidikumba;* Sans. *Lajjalu, Ajalikalika, Namaskari;* Tam. *Totalvadi.*

A very abundant and most troublesome weed in the low country of Ceylon. It is a native of Brazil but has long been naturalized in India and Ceylon.

It is much used in medicine as an alterative and resolvent and is given in cases of corrupted bile and blood. The juice is applied to fistulous sores. According to Ainslie, a decoction of the root of this plant is considered on the Malabar coast to be useful in gravellish complaints. The Vytians of the Coromandel side of India prescribe the leaves and root in cases of piles and fistula; the leaves are given in powder in a little milk to the quantity of two pagodas' weight or more during the day. The root is counted an antidote to cobra poison.

Mucuna pruriens, DC., Eng. *Cowhage;* Sinh. *Vanduru-me, Achari-yapala;* Sans. *Atmagupta, Vanari, Kapikachchu;* Tam. *Pannai-kaali.*

A semi-woody twiner, rather common in the dry and intermediate regions of Ceylon. It is found throughout the Tropics.

It has been used medicinally from the time of Susruta who mentions the seeds as a powerful aphrodisiac. The Bhavaprakasa gives the following directions for their administration :— Take 32 tolas of Mucuna seeds, boil them in four seers of cow's milk till the latter becomes thick. The seeds are now decorticated and pounded, fried in ghee and made into a confection with double their weight of sugar. Dose about a tola (180 grains.) This preparation is claimed to be powerfully aphrodisiac. The root is considered a nervine tonic, and is prescribed in paralysis. In the West Indies, the hairs of the *mucuna* pods are used as a vermifuge to expel ascarides.. A strong infusion of the root, sweetened with honey, is given in South India for cholera.

Phaseolus aconitifolius, Jacq., Eng. *Tapery beans;* Sinh. *Makusthha;*Sans. *Makushtha;* Tam. *Kollu.*

P.Mungo, Linn., Sinh. *Mun;* Sans. *Mudga;* Tam. *Pachchai-payari*, of which there are two varieties, one green and the other yellow, the former being preferred for medicinal purposes.

Phaseolus trilobus, Ait., Sinh. *Munwenna, Bin-me;* Sans. *Mudga-parni;* Tam. *Narippayaru.*

Dolichos biflorus, Linn., Sinh. & Tam. *Kollu;* Sans. *Kulattha.*

Cicer arietinum, Linn., Sinh. *Kadala;* Sans. *Chanaka;* Tam. *Kadalai.*

Vigna luteola, Eng. *Field bean;* Sinh. *Lee-mekaral;* Sans. *Masura*Tam. *Kodeppayaru.*

These pulses are mainly articles of diet. Green *mudga* is considered wholesome and suited to sick persons ; a soup of it is the first article of diet after recovery from acute illness. *Masura, kulattha,* and *makushtha* are considered wholesome and suited for use by convalescents. *Masura* is considered as highly nutritious and useful in bowel complaints ; a poultice of it made with vinegar is an effectual domestic remedy in India for checking the secretion of milk, and reducing swellings of the mammary glands, caused by their distension with milk. A soup made with *kulattha* is said to be antilithic.

Pongamia glabra, Vent., Sinh. *Karanda, Magul-karanda;* Sans. *Karanja, Naktamala;* Tam. *Punku.*

A large tree with a soft grey bark. It is common and grows on banks of streams and rivers near the coast. It is found throughout Tropical Asia.

It is largely used in medicine for many diseases but chiefly in combination with other drugs in dysentery and skin diseases. The root bark is given with other drugs in dysentery : *e.g.*, a useful decoction is made out of ginger, *Cyperus rorundus* (Sinh. *Kalanduru*) and *P.glabra.* A paste made with the seeds along with those of *Cassia tora* and the root of *Sausserea Lappa* is a useful application to skin diseases. The juice of the root is used in cleansing ulcers and closing fistulous sores. The oil is used in itch and rheumatism. It has antiseptic properties and is a useful remedy in scabies, herpes and other cutaneous diseases. *Karanaj* is also an ingredient in several complicated prescriptions for epilepsy and abdominal enlargements. In Tanjore, the juice of the root with coconut milk and lime water is a remedy for gonorrhoea.

The oil obtained from the seeds is known as pongam oil. According to Lepine (Pharm. Journ., (3) XL, 16) the seeds yield 27% of a yellow oil, sp. gr. 0.945, solidifying at 8°. Lewkowitsch obtained by extraction with ether 33.7% of a buttery mass of a dirty yellowish colour which contained 3.05% free fatty acid and 9.22% of unsaponifiable matter. A commercial sample from India gave 0.5% of free fatty acids (in terms of oleic) and 6.9% of unsaponifiable matter.

Psoralea corylifolia, Linn., Sinh. *Bodi;* Sans. *Vakutchi, Lat-kasturika;* Tam. *Karpokarishi.*

A rather rare annual found in the dry region of Ceylon and throughout Peninsular India.

Some works describe the seeds as hot and dry but others as cold and dry, lenitive, fragrant, stimulant and aphrodisiac. They are recommended in leprosy and other cutaneous diseases which are due to a vitiated condition of the blood; they are given internally and applied as a plaster. They are also said to be useful in febrile bilious affections and as an anthelmintic and diuretic. In South India they are used as stomachic and deobstruent.

Kanny Lal Dey (Pharm. Journ. Sept. 1881) strongly recommends the oleo-resinous extract of the seeds diluted with simple unguents as an application in leucoderma :—

"After application for some days the white patches appear to become red or vascular; sometimes a slightly painful sensation is felt. Occasionally some small vesicles or pimples appear, and if these be allowed to remain undisturbed, they dry up, leaving a dark spot of pigmentary matter, which forms as it were a nucleus. From this point as well as from the margin of the patch, pigmentary matters gradually develop, which ultimately coalesce with each other, and thus the whole patch disappears. It is also remarkable that the appearance of fresh patches is arrested by its application."

Pterocarpus Maresupium, Roxb., Eng. *Indian or Malabar Kino;* Sinh. *Gamalu;* Sans. *Pitasala;* Tam. *Venkai.*

A tree with a stout crooked stem, and wide-spreading branches, rather common in the low country of Ceylon, chiefly in the dry and intermediate regions, and also in Southern India. It affords a fine timber, very hard, heavy, dark reddish-brown and durable.

It was not known to the ancient Hindus as a medicine. Its bark exudes a dark-red gum resin, which is known as Indian Kino and is used as a substitute for *Kino Vera.* The peculiar constituent of the gum is kinotannic acid, 70-80%, usually believed to be identical with catechu-tannic acid and distinct from gallo-tannic acid. It is more lenitive than other astringents and is used in the treatment of diarrhoea and pyrosis. The bruised leaves are applied to boils, sores and skin eruptions.

Pterocarpus santalinus, Linn., fil., Eng. *Red Sanders; or Red sandalwood;* Sinh. *Ratsandun;* Sans. *Rakta-chandana;* Tam. *Shen-chandanam,* is a small tree generally met with in the forests of India.

It is regarded as cooling, astringent and tonic and enters into many preparations. It is used as a cooling application to inflamed parts and to the head in headache. As an external application it is supposed to be more powerful than white sandalwood; internally, however, it is less powerful. It is also used as a colouring substance.

In 1870 Weidel exhausted the wood with boiling water containing a little potassium hydroxide and by precipitation with acid obtained a red substance, which on crystallisation with alcohol gave colourless crystals of Santal, $C_8H_6O_3$. $\frac{1}{2}H_2O$. On treatment with alkali the substance yielded protocatechuic and carbonic acids, like piperonal with which it is isomeric. He also obtained a red substance of the formula $C_{14}H_{12}O_4$. In 1870, Franchimont and Sicherer isolated from sandalwood an amorphous principle $C_{17}H_{16}O_6$, m.p., 104°. Three years previous to this Cazeneuve obtained, by extracting with ether, a mixture of sandalwood and lime, a finely crystalline body of the formula $C_{12}H_{10}O_3$. This substance which differed from those already mentioned was a mixture which Cazeneuve and Hugonnenq in 1887 separated into pterocarpin and homopterocarpin, the latter being very soluble in carbon disulphide, whilst the former is soluble only in excess of boiling solvent. Pterocarpine is a white crystalline substance insoluble in cold alcohol and water and strongly laevo-rotatory. Its formula is $C_{10}H_8O_3$, m.p. 152°. Homopterocarpin, $C_{12}H_{12}O_3$, has the same general properties.

Saraca indica, Linn., Eng. *Asoka tree;* Sinh. *Asoka, Hopalu, Diya-ratmal, Diya-ratambala;* San. *Asoka;* Tam. *Ashogan.*

A rather small, much-branched spreading tree, rather common by streams in forests in the low country of Ceylon, India and Malaya. The flowers are very sweet scented; they are at first yellow and become orange and finally red, and are profusely produced for many months.

The bark is strongly astringent and uterine sedative, acting directly on the muscular fibres of the uterus. It has a stimulating effect on the endometrium and the ovarian tissue. It is very useful in menorrhagia due to uterine fibroids. It is also useful in internal bleeding haemorrhoids and haemorrhagic dysentery.

Sesbania aegyptica, Pers., Sinh. *Wel-murunga;* Sans. *Jayanti;* Tam. *Chittakatti,* is a rare woody tree-like herb, found in the dry country of Ceylon and often cultivated throughout the Tropics.

The seeds are described as stimulant, emmenagogue and astringent and useful in checking diarrhoea and excessive menstrual flow, and in reducing enlargements of the spleen. An ointment for itch and other cutaneous eruptions is made from the drug. A poultice of the leaves promotes suppuration of boils and abscesses and absorption of hydrocele and inflammatory swellings.

Sesbania grandiflora, Pers., var Agati grandiflora, Desv., Sinh. *Katuru-murunga;* Sans. *Agastya, Vaka, Sthula-pushpa;* Tam. *Agatti.*

It is cultivated in India and Ceylon, both as a vegetable and as a drug.

The juice of the leaves and flowers is a popular remedy for nasal catarrh and headache when it is sniffed up the nostrils : it causes a copious discharge of fluid and relieves pain and heaviness in the frontal sinuses. The leaves are considered as a very useful remedy for sores. They are regarded also as aperient. They have been found useful in a certain kind of sore-mouth (not sprue), the chief symptom of which is inability to eat hot curries. In such cases the leaves and ox liver cooked form an effective remedy. The bark is given as infusion in the first stages of small-pox and other eruptive fevers. The flowers are cooked and eaten as a vegetable.

Tamarindus Indica, L., Eng. *Tamarind tree;* Sinh. *Siyambala;* Sans. *Tintrani, Amlavriksha;* Tam. *Puli.*

A very commonly planted tree, especially in the dry region.

The unripe fruit is highly acid, the ripe one is less so. The pulp is used in cooking, The ripe fruit of a year or two old is good in atony of the liver, stomach and intestines. It is also useful in preventing or curing scurvy. An agreeable drink known as *amlika-pana* taken when there is loss of appetite, is made by macerating tamarind pulp in water, straining, and adding black pepper, sugar, cloves, camphor and cardamoms to taste. The root bark is astringent and is used in decoctions for dysentery. Powdered seed made into a paste is applied to incipient boils with very good results. The leaves are applied externally in the form of a poultice to inflammatory swellings. The seeds are said to be a good astringent.

Remcaud (J. Pharm. Chim., 1906, vi, 23, 424; Abst., 1906, ii, 483) analysed samples of commercial "crude" and "purified" pulps and compared these with pulp prepared by himself. He found tartaric acid, potassium hydrogen tartrate, invert sugar, sucrose and pectin. The "dry" extract ranged from 62.8 to 73%, ash from 2.8 to 3.2% and total acid calculated as tartaric from 11.7 to 15.8%.

Tephrosia purpurea, Pers., var Galega purpurea, L., Eng. *Purple Tephrosia;* Sinh. *Pila;* Sans. *Saraphunka, Puleehastree, Neelabralakrati;* Tam. *Kolluk-kayvillai.*

A perennial herb, a very common weed in both moist and dry regions of the low country. It is found throughout the Tropics.

It is considered to be diuretic and deobstruent and useful in cough, tightness of the chest and kidney, and is recommended for bilious febrile attacks and obstructions of the liver and spleen. It purifies the blood. The powdered root is smoked in cough, asthma and tightness of the chest. It is given with *cannabis indica* for bleeding piles and with black pepper in cases of gonorrhoea. A decoction of the root is given in dyspepsia and chronic diarrhoea. The root bark ground with black pepper and made into a pill is very beneficial in obstinate colic. An infusion of the seeds is employed as an anthelmintic for children. The oil of the seeds is a specific remedy for scabies, itch and other eruptions. The root is said to be an antidote in snake bite. A congee made with the leaves is recorded to have cured jaundice.

Tephrosia villosa, Pers. var Galega villosa, Sinh. *Boo-pila,* is a very common perennial. It is found in the dry region of Ceylon and in Peninsular India, Tropical Africa and Mauritius. It is given in dropsy.

Clarke and Bannerjee (J. Chem. Soc., 1910, 97, 1833) have isolated and investigated a glucoside from *T.purpurea.* Two pounds of the sun-dried leaves were extracted with 95% alcohol for seven days. The extract was concentrated to a small bulk under atmospheric pressure, poured into water and the green colour removed by extraction with petroleum ether. The dark-brown mother-liquor deposited a copious crop of yellow crystals in about 2½% yield. The substance was crystallised from dilute acetic acid (1:3) and then from dilute alcohol (1:1) or water: yellow needles, m.p., 184-186° (decomp.) were obtained. The pure compound contained water of crystallisation, removable completely at 160°. The air-dried substance has the formula $C_{27}H_{30}O_{16}.\ 3H_2O$; the anhydrous substance is very hygroscopic.

On boiling with 2% aqueous sulphuric acid for six hours the substance gave quercetin and glucose and rhamnose (identified by fractional crystallisation of the phenylosazones). Rhamnose was isolated after fermenting glucose with brewer's yeast. By comparison with a genuine sample, the glucoside was found to be identical with rutin, the glucoside of *Ruta graveoleus.*

Trigonella carniculata, Linn., Sinh. *Pikmal;* Sans. *Malya,* is cultivated as a vegetable. It is similar to spinach. Coumarin is the odorous principle of the plant.

INDEX.

English

A.

B.

C.

Sinhalese

A.

B.

Sanskrit.

A.

Tamil.

A.

C.

D.

English. Sinhalese. Sanskrit. Tamil.

English. Sinhalese. Sanskrit. Tamil.

English.	Sinhalese.	Sanskrit.	Tamil.